THE
Breastfeeding
Survival Guide

THE Breastfeeding Survival Guide

How to feel confident looking after your baby (and yourself)

Danielle Facey

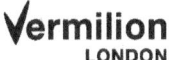
Vermilion
LONDON

VERMILION

UK | USA | Canada | Ireland | Australia
India | New Zealand | South Africa

Vermilion is part of the Penguin Random House group of companies
whose addresses can be found at global.penguinrandomhouse.com

Penguin Random House UK
One Embassy Gardens, 8 Viaduct Gardens, London SW11 7BW

penguin.co.uk
global.penguinrandomhouse.com

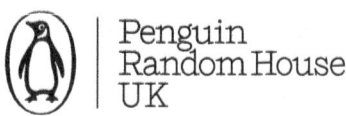

First published by Vermilion in 2025

1

Copyright © Danielle Facey 2025

The moral right of the author has been asserted.

Penguin Random House values and supports copyright. Copyright fuels creativity, encourages diverse voices, promotes freedom of expression and supports a vibrant culture. Thank you for purchasing an authorised edition of this book and for respecting intellectual property laws by not reproducing, scanning or distributing any part of it by any means without permission. You are supporting authors and enabling Penguin Random House to continue to publish books for everyone. No part of this book may be used or reproduced in any manner for the purpose of training artificial intelligence technologies or systems. In accordance with Article 4(3) of the DSM Directive 2019/790, Penguin Random House expressly reserves this work from the text and data mining exception.

Typeset in 10.75/15pt ITC Galliard Pro by Six Red Marbles UK, Thetford, Norfolk
Printed and bound in Great Britain by Clays Ltd, Elcograf S.p.A.

The authorised representative in the EEA is Penguin Random House Ireland,
Morrison Chambers, 32 Nassau Street, Dublin D02 YH68

A CIP catalogue record for this book is available from the British Library

ISBN 9781785045639

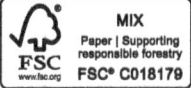

Penguin Random House is committed to a sustainable future for our business, our readers and our planet. This book is made from Forest Stewardship Council® certified paper.

For the boy who made me a mama,
The man who is my home,
And my mother – who stood still so I could fly.

Contents

Introduction — 1
My Story — 2
The Purpose of this Book — 9
How to Use this Book — 13

Chapter One: Beginning Breastfeeding — 17
How Breastfeeding Benefits You — 17
How Breastfeeding Benefits Your Baby — 20
How Breastfeeding Works — 23
Golden Hour — 25
Stimulating Your Milk Supply — 26
Prioritise Rest and Recovery — 32
Coping with Sleep Deprivation — 36
Journalling — 38

Chapter Two: Finding a Rhythm — 41
The Early Weeks: Embracing Flexibility — 41
Feeding in the First Six Weeks — 43
What's Normal? — 45
App or No App? — 47
Night-time Feeding — 49
Finding What Works for You and Your Baby's
    Safety and Comfort — 50
How to Give Yourself Grace as a No-sleep
    Nursing Mama — 52
Global Inspiration — 53
Journal Prompts — 55

How Often Should I Breastfeed My Baby?	58
The Role of Night Feeding	59
Understanding Feeding Patterns and Cluster Feeding	62
Creating a Feeding Log: When Routine Meets Flexibility	62
Understanding Your Own Rhythms	65
Introducing Your Baby to Day and Night Patterns	65
Finding a Rhythm in Breastfeeding: Embracing Adaptability	67

Chapter Three: Managing Your Milk Supply for Nursing and Pumping — 74

Understanding Milk Supply Changes Over Time	74
Understanding Low Supply and Oversupply	75
Managing Low Milk Supply	82
A Balancing Act: Supporting Your Mental Health	86
Potential Causes of True Low Supply	88
Managing your Milk Supply Through Growth Spurts	90
What is Oversupply?	94
Managing Oversupply	96
For Pumping Mothers	102
Navigating the Emotional and Physical Demands of Pumping	104
Journal Prompts	106
The Rewards of Pumping	109
Practical Tips for Managing Pumping	109
Eating to Support Yourself and Your Baby During Breastfeeding	119

Chapter Four: Troubleshooting – Thriving Through the Challenges — 123

Hormonal Changes	124

Oral Ties: Understanding and Addressing Tongue and Lip Ties	124
Coping with Colic	128
Reflux	133
Teething and Breastfeeding	138
Nursing Strikes: When Baby Refuses the Breast	140
Breastfeeding and Sleep Disruptions	144
Nipple Thrush	149
Clogged Ducts and Mastitis	156
Milk Blebs	160
Raynaud's Syndrome and Nipple Blanching	163
Breastfeeding Aversion and Agitation (BAA)	167
Chapter Five: Nurturing Yourself	**172**
Finding Strength Within	172
Recognising the Demands	173
Understanding How Breastfeeding Affects You	174
The Magic of Mother–Infant Attachment	176
Breastfeeding and Postnatal Depression (PND)	176
Understanding Your Constraints and Freedoms	177
Journal Prompts	182
The Power of Music	184
The Magic of Nature	185
Hydration: The Foundation of Wellness	186
Breastfeeding and Alcohol	187
Baby-wearing: The Freedom to Move	190
Tag-team Like a Pro: The Power of Shared Responsibility	192
Epsom Salt Baths: A Simple Escape	194
Stretch and Move: Embracing Gentle Movement and the Wisdom of Yoga	194
The Eight Limbs of Yoga: A Holistic Approach to Self-care	196
Caring for Your Breasts and Your Milk Supply	198

Coping with Unsolicited Advice	200
Self-care in Action	204

Chapter Six: Fuelling Your Breastfeeding — 206

Balanced Diet Tips for Breastfeeding Mothers	207
Nutrient-rich Meal Planning: Invest in Yourself	208
Let Go of Perfectionism	210
Foods to Prioritise and Avoid	211
Hydration for Milk Supply	212
Maintaining Your Energy Levels	212
How to Manage Food Cravings	212
Nourishing Yourself While Breastfeeding	213

Chapter Seven: Breastfeeding and Your Relationships — 215

Your Romantic Relationship	215
How Breastfeeding Hormones Affect You and Your Libido	219
Maintaining Intimacy in the Face of Change	220
Intimacy During Lactation	222
Your Family Dynamics	223
Your Friendships	223
Setting Boundaries with Friends and Family	224
The Evolving Nature of Relationships While Breastfeeding	226

Chapter Eight: Navigating the Transition Back to Work — 227

Journalling Prompts for Returning to Work While Breastfeeding	228
Questions to Ask Your Employer About Pumping at Work	231
How to Breastfeed as a Working Mum	233
How to Deal with Bottle Refusal	237
What is a Freezer Stash?	240

Reverse Cycling: Why It Happens and How to Navigate It 241
You at Work 243
How to Manage a Trip Away from Your Breastfed
    Baby or Toddler 244
Closing Thoughts 248

Chapter Nine: Breastfeeding, Menstruation,
    Fertility and Pregnancy 249
Breastfeeding and Your Period 250
Managing the Return of Your Period 250
Breastfeeding and Your Fertility 251
Journeying Through Pregnancy While
    Breastfeeding 251
Breastfeeding Through Pregnancy: Challenges,
    Changes and Choices 252
Maintaining Your Milk Supply During
    Pregnancy 254
Preparing for Birth While Breastfeeding 256
Compassionate Decision-Making 257
Tandem Breastfeeding 257
How to Tandem Nurse 262

Chapter Ten: How to Stop Breastfeeding 265
Our Weaning Story 266
Child-led Weaning 270
Parent-led Weaning 271
Gentle Weaning: Nourishing and Supporting Young
    Babies and Toddlers Through the Process 274
Navigating the Emotional Transition of Stopping
    Breastfeeding 280

Chapter Eleven: Celebrating Your Breastfeeding
    Journey 285
Honouring Every Breastfeeding Journey 285
Weaning Ceremonies and Traditions 286

The Impact of Breastfeeding – In Any Form	288
Celebrating Every Mother's Choice	289
Words of Wisdom and Affirmations	290
Reflective Journalling and Meditation	294
Final Thoughts	296
References	299
Resources	305
Glossary	307
Index	313
About the Author	323

Introduction

Congratulations on your journey into parenthood! Whether this is your first experience of breastfeeding or chestfeeding, or you are hoping for a different experience this time round, welcome to one of the most remarkable – and often surprisingly complex – journeys in the world. You may have heard from others that nothing can fully prepare you for what lies ahead, and I wholeheartedly agree. But know this: there is so much that you can do to feel more prepared and I am here to offer support, guidance and insights drawn from my own experiences and professional background as The Breastfeeding Mentor.

I trained as a Breastfeeding Peer Support Worker towards the end of my own nursing and pumping journey and was inspired to complete my training as a Breastfeeding Counsellor when I realised just how much need there is for lactation support around the world. This current role built upon previous counsellor training that I'd had during my 13-year teaching career and qualifying very much felt like a full-circle moment. I still feel as passionate as ever about teaching today, but my classroom is typically online and my students are mothers who need just as much tenderness as any troubled teen that I have worked with.

I don't know about you, but I had imagined new motherhood as a blissful whirlwind of coffee dates with my new mum friends, our babies bonding as we did too. Instead, breastfeeding on demand felt like a baptism by fire. I had no idea how much support I would need or how isolated I would feel. Had someone told me then that our breastfeeding journey would last nearly four years, I might have gone into labour all over again . . .

Looking back, I realise that the bigger issue was my unrealistic expectations of motherhood in general. Though I had spent time with friends and family who had babies, my visits usually lasted only a few hours and I was focussed primarily on cuddling their tiny newborn. I now understand that many parents are reluctant to openly discuss the challenges of parenthood with non-parents, either for fear of judgment or because they know it is too difficult to truly comprehend. In my case, I also acknowledge that I may also have been deaf to some of my friends' complaints about the realities of parenting due to my experience with baby loss.

I am hoping that this book sparks a change in the narrative that we should only share the positive aspects of breastfeeding and new motherhood with expecting parents. For me, toxic positivity surrounding nursing and pumping made me feel like there was something wrong with me for finding it so difficult. Through the wonders of social media – for all its misgivings – I know that this is also the case for many mothers around the world. So, let's keep it real – for all our sakes. Let us discuss the myriad benefits of breastfeeding, whilst also acknowledging the reality of the challenges, too.

My Story

'Breast may well be best, but it might also kill me in the process . . .' That was the phrase running through my mind as I entered the milk-soaked world of breastfeeding.

I had an incredibly traumatic birthing experience – perhaps you did too. It was far from the unmedicated water birth I had envisioned, and it left me feeling powerless and like a failure. That birth story, coupled with my previous experience of baby loss, made me more determined than ever to breastfeed our rainbow baby boy. The perfectionist within piled on the pressure for me to do everything in my power to redeem myself as a mother. Looking back, I wish I'd have given myself even an ounce of the love and grace that I so deserved.

It took four days before my son was able to latch onto me. Until then, I hand-expressed colostrum (the first milk your breasts produce) day and night to feed him, using tiny syringes. I had expected breastfeeding to be challenging but I had no idea just how much hands-on support I would need in those early days. I owe our breastfeeding success to the ever-patient love of my life, as well as a rather harassed lactation-trained midwife and a dear friend who impressed upon me the importance of not leaving the hospital before I felt confident in my son's latch.

After a rocky start, I was beyond grateful to be able to exclusively nurse our baby boy. I hoped we could follow the World Health Organisation's recommendation of breastfeeding exclusively for six months, then alongside solid foods for two years or beyond . . . That was until we settled into the reality of breastfeeding on demand. During the first few months, our son woke every two to three hours to nurse. While my Health Visitor assured me this was completely normal, I couldn't help but wonder how sustainable it would be. How could I possibly make it to six months of exclusive breastfeeding if that meant just a few hours of broken sleep each night? How was I supposed to care for myself – eat well, exercise, or maintain any semblance of a social life? Where was the guidance on how to take care of myself whilst I was breastfeeding?

So often, breastfeeding is depicted as natural and intuitive, whilst the reality is that for many parents, these experiences can be fraught with challenges – physical, emotional and societal. I have worked closely with parents who felt immense pressure, guilt or even failure when things didn't go as planned, and I want to stress that your mental health during this time is as important as your baby's nourishment. When we thrive, our children can too. This book exists to help you navigate those challenges, equipping you with tools and support so you feel empowered, not judged, in your feeding journey.

I am a trained yoga and meditation teacher, and this also informs my work with breastfeeding mums. Yoga's philosophy and practices are not only about physical postures but also about cultivating mindfulness, compassion and balance. I truly understand the profound connection between the body and mind, and how supporting one can nurture the other.

For breastfeeding mothers, these principles are invaluable. One of the first things I focus on when working with new clients is helping mothers cultivate a calm and supportive space for themselves, which ties into the yogic principle of Yamas – moral disciplines – encouraging non-violence (Ahimsa) towards oneself. This means being gentle with your body, acknowledging the physical and emotional challenges that may arise during breastfeeding and offering yourself compassion through this demanding time. I focus specifically on how yogic practices and meditation can support your breastfeeding journey at various points throughout this book and with a special focus in Chapters Three and Five (see pages 74 and 172).

For me, this journey is more than professional; it is deeply personal. My own experiences of motherhood, baby loss and healing have profoundly shaped the way I view and approach breastfeeding. Over the years, I have had the privilege of supporting thousands of parents around the world through the challenges of breastfeeding and chestfeeding. From providing new mothers with in-person, hands-on support as a Peer Helper and coaching mums through their return to work, to holding their hands when they stop breastfeeding, this work has shone a light on how truly transformative knowledge and unconditional support can be. I get to see every day how, when mothers are empowered to feed their babies on their own terms, they are less anxious and more self-assured. They doubt themselves and their incredible capabilities less and they allow themselves to seek the help and guidance that they need without guilt or shame. This has a transformative effect on their lives and those of their families.

This guide embraces and empowers all feeding journeys. While I'll primarily use the term breastfeeding throughout, this book is just as much for those who are chestfeeding or feeding in other ways, recognising that every journey is unique. I also use the terms *mother* and *parent* interchangeably. No matter how you feed your baby, you deserve to feel supported, seen and understood.

It's important to acknowledge that while some of you may be breastfeeding exclusively, nursing your baby at the breast, some of you might be pumping or expressing. Some of you may be doing a combination, feeding your baby your milk (whether pumped or at the breast) alongside donor milk or formula. The reasons for these choices are as varied as the parents who make them. While I understand why the phrase 'breast is best' exists, I truly believe that every parent is doing their best with the circumstances they face. This book is written to empower your choices – whether they are made out of necessity, preference or both.

At the same time, the phrase 'fed is best' may also be problematic. While it's true that 'fed' is a non-negotiable requirement, the phrase can unintentionally undermine breastfeeding and lend undue support to formula use without recognising the wider context. Formula is a life-saving food that empowers millions of parents to feed their babies, yet the formula industry's aggressive and unethical promotion of such slogans has a troubling global history. For me, 'empowered and supported is best' – though I admit, it doesn't have quite the same catchy ring!

I also recognise the need to make distinctions between exclusively breastfeeding, exclusively pumping or mixed feeding. I write this book also for the mothers who are open to the flexibility of pumping but find that their bodies don't respond well to it or their babies won't take a bottle. There are also babies who can't latch, and the topic of nursing may carry a deep sense of grief if this is your experience. As with so very many aspects of parenting, ultimately, we all want to do right by our children, our families and ourselves. With that in mind, this book is for anyone who lactates or hopes to do so – in any capacity.

The Breastfeeding Survival Guide contains the advice I wish I'd received during those blissfully unaware weeks before giving birth and the sleep-deprived months that followed. This book is for *all* breastfeeding journeys – whether you breastfeed for three days, three months or three years. It is also for parents who combination feed, offering breast milk alongside formula. Continuing to breastfeed while supplementing is not a failure; it is a valid and empowering way to meet your baby's needs while also caring for yourself. If more parents felt confident combining breastfeeding with formula when necessary, I believe far fewer would stop breastfeeding altogether. My hope is that this book will help you feel empowered to breastfeed in a way that works for *you*.

Alongside my yoga background, my approach to breastfeeding support is rooted in my experience as a teacher of English and Psychology. I understand that the transition to parenthood is immense – you might be feeling it's far more profound than society acknowledges – and it is a steep learning curve.

I earned a Master's Degree in Psychology in 2017 to better understand myself and the minds I was helping to shape. My research focussed specifically on educational transitions and their significant impact on children's well-being and success. This understanding has influenced my professional practice and shaped my parenting journey – and it's central to the guidance I offer here.

During the first global lockdown in 2020, as a fragile and isolated new mother, I learned about the permanent transition of matrescence. Coined in the 1970s by anthropologist Dana Raphael, matrescence describes the physical, psychological and emotional changes a person experiences when becoming a mother. The term combines 'maternity' and 'adolescence', reflecting the magnitude of the hormonal, cognitive and emotional transformations that occur during this period. At the time, I had just returned to my full-time role as a teacher after maternity leave – barely a month before the global pandemic struck. A few weeks later, I collapsed from sheer exhaustion while attempting to do the weekly food shop.

Looking back it seems unimaginable that I believed I could return seamlessly and without support to my role as an English and Psychology teacher, alongside my duties as a boarding housemistress. My return to work coincided with the developmental peak of my son's separation anxiety, which meant he woke every hour overnight to nurse and reconnect with me after my 14-hour workdays. During my back-to-work meetings, I mentioned how wakeful my son had become and explained that I was still breastfeeding. The response from my managers? 'Time to cut the cord!'

When I requested flexible working hours during that same meeting, I was told I had every right to submit a request but that it would only be considered if it served the best interests of the business. Needless to say, the implication was that it didn't.

My family doctor was no help. She sympathised with me but ultimately had no advice beyond her own experiences of motherhood. Her recommendation? 'Just go away for the weekend, and hopefully, when you return, he'll be so mad at you that he won't want to nurse anymore. That's what I did!'

Anxious and overwhelmed, I reached out to fellow new mothers and friends for advice on navigating this transition. Almost universally, I was met with the same suggestions: stop breastfeeding and sleep train your baby so that he 'learns' to fall asleep independently. Neither of these solutions aligned with my instincts or our parenting style. I simply could not reconcile leaving our rainbow baby boy to cry himself to sleep alone at night.

The situation felt impossible.

You may have felt the same: wanting desperately to continue to breastfeed, but with no clue how to find a way through? This book is designed to hold you by the hand and help you make choices that sit right with your body, heart and mind.

Breastfeeding meant the world to me. After a previous pregnancy loss and a traumatic birth experience, it was a deeply healing part of my journey. My son adored nursing, too – it brought him comfort, connection and nourishment and was the only guaranteed way to help him fall asleep at any time of day or night. The thought of abruptly stopping felt unnecessary, but also emotionally unbearable for us both.

It was just a few weeks after my physical and emotional breakdown that *The Breastfeeding Mentor* was born. However, the journey to that point began almost a decade before my first social media post.

In the summer of 2014, after a decade of marriage, I felt ready to start a family with my then-husband. Despite having Polycystic Ovary Syndrome (PCOS) – a hormonal disorder and leading cause of infertility – I was fortunate to fall pregnant after just a few months of trying. I felt like the luckiest woman in the world.

I had a scan at just seven weeks of pregnancy and proudly shared the ultrasound image with our nearest and dearest. But around midnight on the day I turned 12 weeks pregnant – the so-called 'safe zone' – I heartbreakingly lost our baby. Anyone who has experienced grief knows it leaves a hole in your heart that can never be filled. Yet, with time and healing, you learn to live alongside that loss. I share this story because I know that my drive and determination to breastfeed my rainbow baby boy was born from this heartache. I felt, in my core, that I had failed as a mother in the most absolute way. I had failed to bring my baby safely into the world.

For anyone reading this who has experienced the loss of a baby in any form, I want you to know: *I see you. I feel you. I am you.* I believe my lost baby was a girl, and my memories of loving her remain as vivid as ever. When I allow myself to think about her, the pain still feels as raw as it did on that cold summer morning. Yet, knowing that she spent her entire life in my embrace gives me some comfort.

There's also a small scientific solace I have drawn from a phenomenon called microchimerism. Research suggests that some of a baby's cells remain within the mother's body after pregnancy. These 'healing cells' migrate into the mother's bloodstream, sometimes staying for years, where they may even play a role in physical and emotional healing. For me, this discovery has been a profound source of connection and strength. It comforts me deeply to know that a part of my baby, though physically gone, still lives within me.

The Purpose of this Book

For many parents, feeding their baby becomes a defining part of early parenthood – one that often evokes a mixture of joy, frustration, pride and doubt. It is an intimate journey that is as unique as your bond with your baby. The reality is that no two feeding experiences look the same, and that's okay. What matters most is finding a way to nourish your baby that works for *you* – one that respects both your physical needs and your emotional well-being.

You have likely read numerous baby books – those that offer guidance on everything from bathing your newborn to ensuring the ideal nursery temperature, and some even go as far as explaining the colour, consistency and frequency of your baby's first poos! However, what they often overlook is how to care for *yourself* while you are caring for your baby. This book is for *you*.

For some, breastfeeding may feel natural from the start, and if this is your experience, that's wonderful! However, even for those who find it comes more easily, it's important to recognise that breastfeeding is still a learning process for both you and your baby. It's completely normal and more common for it to take time to find your flow. For many – myself included – breastfeeding can feel incredibly challenging in the beginning. No matter your experience, remember that breastfeeding is a journey that often requires patience and practice before it feels anywhere near the instinctive, bonding experience often portrayed in the media. I share this information not to terrify you but to normalise the fact that breastfeeding, although natural, is rarely easy. In fact, more often than not it takes a significant amount of time, energy, effort, practice and determination to find your rhythm and confidence. But remember, we can do hard things – particularly with support.

If breastfeeding is presenting challenges which are making you doubt yourself, I strongly encourage you to seek help in person from a qualified International Board Certified Lactation Consultant (IBCLC), a breastfeeding counsellor or a peer support group. These professionals and networks are trained to guide you through every aspect of breastfeeding, offering invaluable support tailored to your needs. As a breastfeeding peer helper, breastfeeding counsellor and with my online services as *The Breastfeeding Mentor*, I've supported many mothers through the ups and downs of their breastfeeding journeys, helping them to trust their instincts and believe in themselves. Seeking support is not a badge of shame, it is a sign of your innate understanding that you deserve all the help in the world to breastfeed if it is important to you.

Too often, new parents feel unsupported or isolated, not because others don't care, but because of a lack of understanding. Well-meaning, unsolicited advice from family and friends can undermine your confidence. My goal is to empower you with information and support, helping you navigate the physiological, practical and societal challenges of breastfeeding with greater confidence. This book is a resource for *you*, offering encouragement as you tackle the unique challenges of new motherhood – especially during those early days when your baby seems permanently attached to the breast. You are not alone, and by trusting yourself and seeking support when needed, you *will* find your way.

We'll explore questions you may not have considered yet, such as: How do you survive on only three or four hours of broken sleep each night? How do you find time to shower when your newborn won't let you put them down for more than 30 seconds? And, during the rare 15 minutes of me-time that you may get each day, how can you feel like *yourself* again, rather than a milk machine? These were questions I hadn't thought to ask before giving birth, but fear not – knowledge is power. Understanding these challenges before they arise helps you prepare for them. This book provides practical tips to help new parents do just that, allowing you to embrace and enjoy breastfeeding – and motherhood – in all its bleary-eyed, milk-soaked glory.

It is important to acknowledge that breastfeeding challenges can sometimes feel overwhelming, and there can be immense pressure to meet societal expectations. Many parents feel a sense of failure when faced with difficulties, especially if their journey doesn't match the idealised images often portrayed. Once more, I want to emphasise that your mental health during this time is incredibly important. Studies show that around one-fifth of new mothers experience postnatal depression and the emotional toll can be even greater if feeding struggles are involved. This is an area I work closely on with parents, helping them navigate both the practical challenges of feeding and the emotional hurdles that can arise.

Sadly, not every parent who wishes to breastfeed is able to. It's estimated that 1–5 per cent of women are physiologically unable to produce enough milk to exclusively breastfeed. So why are breastfeeding rates in the UK and US among the lowest in the world? Between 2020 and 2024, up to 85 per cent of mothers in the UK initiated breastfeeding, but only around a quarter of mothers were doing so exclusively at six months. Median breastfeeding duration across the UK was around 39 days. In the US, 83 per cent of mothers started breastfeeding; by six months, only 25 per cent were exclusively breastfeeding.

When I learned that eight out of ten mothers stop breastfeeding earlier than they had planned, I felt deeply saddened. Why do so many parents stop breastfeeding when they initially want to continue? A 2019 literature review revealed that the primary reasons were perceived low milk supply and breast or nipple pain. For me, and the mums I work with every day, the lack of support surrounding nursing and pumping was not due to malice, but to ignorance. As a new mother, just like my clients, I simply didn't know what to expect or what to do when things seemed to be going wrong and neither did my well-meaning family and friends.

I have written this book for you, for me, my sisters, friends and any mother who needs guidance when support is limited. I am passionate about ensuring that every mother feels empowered to breastfeed for as long as she chooses. Having survived the baptism of fire that is the fourth trimester (and beyond!), I feel privileged to have nursed our son for three years and nine months. I am eternally grateful that our journey ended when we were both ready. No matter your journey – whether short or long, exclusive or combined – you are not alone. This book is here to help you feel confident, supported and empowered *every* step of the way.

How to Use this Book

Breastfeeding is a deeply personal and transformative journey, but it isn't a one-size-fits-all experience. This book is here to be your guide and companion throughout every stage, offering the tools, guidance and support to help you thrive while breastfeeding, whether you're in the early stages or approaching the time to wean. Think of it as your personal breastfeeding encyclopedia, where you can dip in whenever you need advice, comfort or inspiration.

You can start wherever you need to, whether you're facing your first latch or navigating the challenges of breastfeeding beyond infancy. This isn't a book that requires reading cover to cover, but a collection of insights, tools and practices that will meet you exactly where you are. It is meant to be a living, breathing resource, giving you practical advice, emotional support and empowering you to find a rhythm that works for you and your precious baby.

Each chapter is designed to give you the confidence to make informed decisions about your breastfeeding journey. With reflective journal prompts, breathing exercises, affirmations and mindfulness practices, you'll find interactive tools that help you remain grounded, calm and supported. It's so important that you nourish your own body and soul as well as your child's.

Here's how you can use my book:

- **Jump to the chapter you need:** If you're struggling with latch issues or you're dealing with teething and nursing strikes, simply go straight to the relevant chapter. The book is meant to serve as a flexible resource for when you need advice or strategies on specific challenges.

- **Reflect and recharge:** In addition to practical advice, each chapter contains journal prompts, visualisations or breathing exercises that you can return to whenever you need emotional and mental support. These are designed to help you pause, reflect and care for yourself. It's about nourishing your physical, mental and emotional well-being throughout the breastfeeding journey.

- **Interactive support:** As you read, you'll encounter mantras and meditations that can help you centre your mind and calm your central nervous system – both of which support milk production and your emotional well-being. These tools can be used at any time, especially during moments when you feel overwhelmed or need grounding.

Your journey is unique and I'm here to support you on that. A practical, compassionate companion to help you face each challenge with calm, patience and confidence. The tools, tips and reflections within are designed to make breastfeeding easier, more fulfilling and full of grace. Remember, you're not alone – through the words on these pages, you are connected to me and the global Breastfeeding Mentor community. It takes a village, and often we feel a sense of complete lack of that support that we expect to have – support from other people in your own family, the relatives who might have breastfed and have advice to give. Sometimes, we are lucky enough to truly feel seen and supported by those in our family, our mothers/mothers-in-law/sisters/grandmothers. But too often, there may be figures who clash with our hoped-for style, we may feel judged or an absence of their empathy and guidance? Generational wisdom that could be such a gift, can often feel instead like a hindrance. And this is the exact gap that this book seeks to fill. Stand on the shoulders of the giants who have come before you and tap into the generational wisdom that so many of us yearn for as we breastfeed. I want to support you from your first feed to your last.

Welcome to your breastfeeding journey – you've got this.

CHAPTER ONE

Beginning Breastfeeding

Beyond helping you form a deep attachment, breastfeeding provides significant health benefits for both you and your baby. This chapter will offer you clear, evidence-based information about those benefits and take a look at some common myths that may be influencing your thoughts about nursing your baby. There can be so many misconceptions and societal attitudes surrounding breastfeeding that may discourage or confuse new mothers and parents.

It's my firm belief that with the right support, guidance, patience and understanding, a positive breastfeeding experience is absolutely within reach for you, although journey may not be straightforward and there will likely be challenges along the way. Research shows that around eight out of ten mothers in the UK begin breastfeeding, but only a small percentage continue to breastfeed exclusively by six months. For me this shows a real need for more support and information to help new parents breastfeed as they hope to. In this chapter, we'll lay the foundation for a golden start, focussing on the key principles that will give you the best possible beginning, and set you up for the confidence and resilience to overcome anything that is thrown into your path.

How Breastfeeding Benefits You

Let's begin by celebrating the advantages of breastfeeding. Incredibly, research indicates that for every year that you breastfeed, your risk of developing breast cancer decreases. A 2021 review supports this, revealing that mothers who breastfeed for more than 12 months experience a 26 per cent lower risk of breast cancer. Comparing breastfeeding durations, women who breastfed for 12–23 months had a 66.3 per cent reduction in breast cancer risk compared to those who breastfed for 0–11 months. This reduction increases significantly for longer breastfeeding durations, with an 87.4 per cent reduction for those breastfeeding 24–35 months and an impressive 94 per cent reduction for those in the 36–47 months range. If, like me, breast cancer runs in your family, it can feel comforting to know that the act of nursing or pumping for your baby can reduce your risk of developing the disease.

Recent international studies provide encouraging news for mothers who have survived breast cancer. These studies reveal that breastfeeding after breast cancer does not increase the risk of cancer recurrence or new breast cancers. If this applies to you, this research marks a significant milestone, affirming that you can choose to breastfeed without fear. For many women, this opens the door to a fulfilling breastfeeding experience after their cancer journey, promoting a sense of connection with their baby while supporting their own health.

Studies have shown that breastfeeding significantly lowers your risk of developing ovarian cancer, a disease often difficult to detect early and frequently diagnosed in its later stages. One study revealed that women who breastfed for at least six months had a 30 per cent lower risk of developing ovarian cancer compared to those who never breastfed. It's believed that breastfeeding suppresses ovulation, reducing exposure to certain hormones associated with ovarian cancer development.

Breastfeeding also provides significant cardiovascular benefits, reducing the risk of hypertension and heart disease. A recent meta-analysis concluded that breastfeeding women had a 9 per cent lower risk of developing cardiovascular disease and a 12 per cent reduction in the risk of hypertension, likely due to the body's physiological adjustments to the demands of milk production and the relaxing influence of prolactin and oxytocin. These hormone shifts support heart health by lowering blood pressure and improving cholesterol profiles, which contribute to better cardiovascular outcomes overall. Breastfeeding, then, is more than just providing for your baby's needs – it's a gift to yourself as well, one that strengthens your heart, both emotionally and physically.

Incredibly, breastfeeding has been linked to improved bone health later in life, reducing the risk of osteoporosis. Lactation prompts our bodies to release calcium stored in our bones to support milk production, initially decreasing bone density. However, this loss is temporary and post-weaning, your body undergoes a remarkable 'rebuilding' phase that often results in stronger, denser bones. In fact, a 2020 study highlighted that women who breastfed for more than 12 months had a 15 per cent lower risk of osteoporosis compared to those who did not breastfeed, with additional benefits observed in those who breastfed multiple children.

It is truly awe-inspiring that emerging research is exploring the neuroprotective effects of breastfeeding, including a reduced risk of Alzheimer's disease in breastfeeding mums. A recent long-term study found a correlation between breastfeeding and a 23 per cent lower risk of developing cognitive decline and dementia, potentially due to the lasting effects of hormonal balance, improved cardiovascular health and other biochemical responses associated with lactation. These remarkable benefits really underscore breastfeeding's holistic impact, showing that this natural practice contributes to our physical and mental health in ways we are only just beginning to fully understand.

A message that I will reiterate throughout this book is that breastfeeding is good for you, mama, for as long as it works for you, your family and your unique circumstances.

How Breastfeeding Benefits Your Baby

Breastfeeding is more than just providing nutrition; it is a powerful way of nurturing your baby physically, mentally and emotionally. Breast milk is a living fluid which adapts to support your little one's changing needs, supporting every aspect of their health and well-being. It is truly a wonder, and so are you.

Breast milk is often called 'liquid gold' and for good reason. Packed with everything your baby needs to grow and thrive, it's a perfect blend of proteins, fats, carbohydrates, vitamins and minerals, all tailored specifically for their individual and evolving needs. These nutrients work together like little building blocks, supporting not just their growth, but their brain development too[x]. Two of the superstar components in breast milk, DHA (omega-3) and ARA (omega-6), are essential fatty acids that are vital for your baby's nerve and eye development. DHA is especially crucial for forming brain synapses and cell membranes, which directly influences your little one's cognitive abilities. Breast milk is truly a natural miracle, packed into every drop.

Cognitive growth is all about those amazing abilities your child will develop over time – from learning to speak to improving memory and focus. Breastfeeding's positive impact on brain development can last well into childhood, helping your little one with everything from socialising to excelling at school and beyond. It's like giving them the gift of a brighter future, one feed at a time.

Your baby's immune system is particularly vulnerable in the first months of life, making them more susceptible to infections and illnesses. Breast milk provides powerful immunological support by transferring antibodies and white blood cells from you to your baby, offering passive immunity that protects against common infections. Studies show that breastfed babies are far less likely to suffer from things like respiratory infections, tummy troubles and ear infections compared to babies who are formula-fed. It's just another way that your milk is working its magic, offering your little one that extra layer of protection and keeping them healthier for longer. Writing as a mother who had a nine-month old when the global pandemic struck, it felt incredible to be able to bolster my son's immune system with my own during uncertain times.

Breast milk is packed with enzymes and other goodness that help to regulate your baby's immune system and keep inflammation in check. When you breastfeed, that beautiful skin-to-skin contact isn't just comforting – it's also incredibly beneficial for your baby's gut health, transferring those all-important healthy bacteria that are key for their developing immune system. Plus, this strong start helps lower the risk of allergies, asthma and chronic conditions, giving your baby the very best foundation for lifelong health.

Breastfeeding isn't just about the physical health benefits – it's also about nurturing your baby's emotional well-being. That closeness, the eye contact and the simple act of holding your baby during feeding creates a deep sense of security and trust between you both. And let's not forget the wonder that is oxytocin, the 'love hormone' which flows through you during breastfeeding, helping you both feel calm and connected. This bonding time isn't just comforting – it lays the foundation for a secure attachment, helping your child develop emotional resilience and the ability to form strong, positive relationships as they grow. Breastfeeding nurtures not just your baby's body, but their heart and mind too.

The deep bond formed through breastfeeding can shape your child's emotional landscape in profound ways. Secure attachment, nurtured during these tender moments, is linked to improved social skills, better emotional regulation and lower anxiety. Toddlers and young children who have a strong attachment tend to be more confident in exploring their world and engaging with others. This sense of security helps them build lasting relationships and develop empathy, making it easier for them to adapt socially as they grow. It's a powerful foundation that continues to support them as they learn how to navigate life and connect with the people around them.

Breastfeeding benefits stretch far beyond the early months and years, with impressive long-term health effects. Studies suggest that breastfeeding even offers protective effects against chronic conditions like obesity, type 2 diabetes and heart disease later in life. This could be due to breast milk's unique ability to promote healthy metabolic processes in infancy, influencing everything from weight regulation to insulin sensitivity. By nurturing your baby's metabolism with breast milk, from the start, you're setting the stage for them to have a healthier future.

Alongside all this, breastfeeding helps establish a healthy gut microbiome, which plays a key role in your child's long-term health. The beneficial bacteria found in breast milk support the development of balanced gut flora, which is crucial for a strong immune system and reduced inflammation. A thriving gut can help protect against many conditions related to inflammation and metabolic issues, offering yet another reason to cherish the lasting health benefits of breastfeeding.

Even beyond infancy, breastfeeding continues to offer tailored benefits for toddlers and young children. As they grow, they continue to receive immunological, emotional and nutritional support from nursing. While societal attitudes towards breastfeeding older children vary, research shows that continued breastfeeding supports both physical and psychological health well into toddlerhood and beyond. For toddlers, breast milk is a valuable source of high-quality nutrients, particularly during times when their appetite is notoriously unpredictable due to growth spurts or developmental changes. Rich in protein, fats and essential vitamins, it's the ideal complement to their ever-changing diet.

Whether through nursing or pumping – breastfeeding is a wonderful source of nutrition and connection for you and your baby, as long as it feels right for you both. There's no one-size-fits-all answer and only you can decide what works best for your family. If anyone feels the need to pass judgment on your breastfeeding journey, quite frankly, they should mind their own tits!

How Breastfeeding Works

When your baby latches on and begins to suckle, it's not just a physical action – it's a communication system that activates your body's hormone release. First up, your brain gets the message that it's time to produce milk, and in response, it releases prolactin. This hormone is your milk-maker; it stimulates special cells in your breast called lactocytes. The more your baby feeds, the more prolactin is released, making sure you produce enough milk for their growing needs.

As your baby suckles and stimulates your nipple, your brain releases oxytocin. Not only does oxytocin have a calming, soothing effect on both you and your baby, but it's also the key hormone that makes your milk flow. Inside your breasts are small storage spaces where the milk collects. When oxytocin is triggered by your baby's suckling, the milk is squeezed into the ducts, ready for your baby to drink.

Oxytocin does so much more than just help your milk flow – this beautiful hormone also deepens the bond between you and your little one. It promotes feelings of closeness, trust and connection, making those quiet moments of feeding even more intimate and nurturing for both of you. It's all part of the powerful dance of hormones that makes breastfeeding such a special, rewarding experience. It is worth noting that not every nursing or pumping parent experiences this rush of love – you can read more about nursing aversion or Dysphoric Milk Ejection Reflex (D-MER) in Chapter Three (see page 74).

When oxytocin is released, you might feel a wave of relaxation, sometimes a little sleepy, and often a deep sense of love and warmth. It's what makes those moments of breastfeeding so special for many – it's not just nourishment but a true bonding experience, where you and your baby are emotionally and physically connected.

These hormones work in harmony. Prolactin is responsible for ensuring you have enough milk to feed your baby and oxytocin is the hormone that makes sure milk flows when your baby needs it. It's all part of how your body is designed to support your little one, and once you both find your rhythm, it can truly feel like the most rewarding and natural thing in the world.

I was personally taken aback by how powerfully these fundamental breastfeeding hormones affected me. I'll never forget the first time my son latched on at around 3am on his fourth day earthside. A wave of love, warmth and drowsiness washed over me, from the crown of my head to the tips of my toes. It was such a palpable and intense sensation that I struggled to stay upright and awake. I only wish I had known then what I know now about safe bed-sharing and co-sleeping practices – but more on that, as well as what to do if your baby isn't latching without support, in a later chapter (see page 50).

How to Get off to the Best Possible Start

Once breastfeeding is well-established, it can feel like the fuzzy, warm spiritual experience we might hope for. However, the early days may bring discomfort as you and your baby get used to the skill and rhythm of it. It's important to remember that breastfeeding *shouldn't* be excruciatingly painful. If you're experiencing unbearable pain, it's a sign that something is not quite right; seek urgent face-to-face support from an International Board Certified Lactation Consultant (IBCLC), peer supporter or breastfeeding counsellor.

Golden Hour

The first hour after birth, often referred to as 'Golden Hour' is a critical window for establishing breastfeeding and supporting your newborn's early development. During this time, skin-to-skin contact between mother and baby can significantly enhance the release of oxytocin. Oxytocin release helps regulate both yours and your baby's temperature and heart rate, which helps to stabilise your newborn's early environment.

Uninterrupted skin-to-skin contact immediately after birth helps to kickstart your baby learning to breastfeed and is associated with higher rates of breastfeeding continuation. Ideally, soon after birth your baby should be placed directly onto your chest without interference – eager grandparents can wait – for at least an hour. This encourages your newborn to naturally seek your boobs and begin to feed. Some babies even make their own way to the breast after being placed on their mother's chest after birth, by doing what is known as a 'breast crawl'. The practice of being undisturbed immediately after birth can also support your milk supply by sending strong signals to your body to begin milk production in response to your baby's feeding cues.

Skin-to-skin contact isn't just something to embrace during the Golden Hour – it's something to continue in the early days, weeks and even months after birth. It's an incredibly powerful practice that helps regulate your newborn's temperature, stabilise their blood glucose and improve oxygenation and respiratory rates, too. For you, skin-to-skin contact can also have a wonderful impact on your milk supply. It boosts prolactin levels, the hormone responsible for milk production, helping to strengthen and support your breastfeeding journey.

However, it's important to acknowledge that not everyone's birth experience is as smooth or straightforward as hoped. If you or your baby faced challenges after birth – whether it was due to illness, a Caesarean or birth trauma – it's completely okay. You may not have been able to hold your baby right away and that's alright. I couldn't either. This doesn't mean breastfeeding can't be successfully established. Every journey is unique, and while the hormonal domino effect of birth can be delicate, it's never too late to start. Our bodies are remarkably adaptable. If you've had a more challenging birth experience, as I did, please give yourself some grace. Trust that with the right support, patience and time, your body can still respond beautifully to the bonding process.

Even fathers and other supportive family members can be involved in skin-to-skin contact, helping to lay a strong foundation for family bonding, emotional support and those precious early connections. No matter how your birth unfolds, there's always an opportunity to create these meaningful moments with your baby.

Stimulating Your Milk Supply

In ideal circumstances, you'll receive support early on to help your baby latch on in those first few hours after birth to get your milk flowing. The delivery of your placenta plays a pivotal role in this process. Once the placenta is delivered, your body experiences a drop in pregnancy hormones, particularly progesterone, which has been keeping your milk production in check. This drop signals to your body that it's time to start making milk, thanks to prolactin, the hormone that now takes centre stage.

Your breasts actually begin producing milk long before birth; from around the third month of pregnancy, your body starts producing colostrum, the thick, nutrient-rich first milk your baby will drink in those early days.

Your milk supply begins in earnest usually within the first few days after birth. It's important to note that this transition doesn't always happen immediately and it's perfectly normal for your milk to come in gradually. This is especially true if you've had a Caesarean section, as I did. The early days can sometimes feel unpredictable, and that's okay! Rest assured, your body is working hard behind the scenes and each feed, pump or hand expression session helps increase your milk supply.

In the meantime, your newborn's tummy is only around the size of a cherry, holding between five and seven millilitres (one teaspoon) of milk when they are first born. It will gradually grow to around the size of an egg after a month, holding up to 150ml (5oz) of milk. With this in mind, don't worry about producing millilitres and millilitres of milk from the moment your baby is born. Give your milk supply time to adapt and grow with your baby. Research suggests that it is feeding frequency that matters more than anything in those early days.

When your baby begins nursing, their sucking triggers the release of more prolactin, creating a beautiful feedback loop that encourages your body to produce more milk. This is why early and frequent breastfeeding is so important – whether it's at the breast or through hand expression if your baby is struggling to latch. These early moments of milk removal are crucial for your body to recognise the demand for milk and respond accordingly, helping to establish a full milk supply.

If colostrum is not being regularly removed, your body won't receive the signal it needs to ramp up production.

This can lead to a low milk supply, which is one of the reasons why 'the formula trap' can be so challenging. When formula is introduced early on, your baby's belly may be filled, but they're not stimulating your milk production. As a result your body doesn't increase milk output and this can lead to frustration, as your baby may become unsettled at the breast.

I want to be clear that this is not to discourage you from using formula if that's part of your feeding plan – every family's journey is unique, and you should absolutely do what feels right for you. However, it's important to understand that introducing formula during the early days may make it a bit trickier to establish your milk supply. By focussing on breastfeeding or expressing as often as possible, you'll be giving your body the best chance to establish a robust milk supply, setting the foundation for a successful breastfeeding journey – even alongside formula. It's a process that takes patience and support, but your body knows exactly what to do – it just needs time and space to adjust.

One of the most valuable pieces of advice I received early on was to have my son's latch checked – repeatedly – before leaving the hospital. This may seem like a small thing, but for me, it made all the difference. Thanks to a wonderful (though overworked) lactation-trained midwife on the ward and a breastfeeding unit just a few miles away, I was able to ensure my son's latch was deep and comfortable. This support meant I knew what to look for and how to adjust both myself and my baby if his latch wasn't quite right at the start of a feed. Being able to make these adjustments early on helped us avoid many of the challenges that often arise in those first few days postpartum.

Unfortunately, not everyone has access to immediate support, which is why it's so important to know what to look for and when to seek help.

A Note on Tongue Ties

The topic of tongue ties has recently sparked significant media attention, with some reports questioning the rising number of infants undergoing the corrective procedure, known as a frenectomy. While there has indeed been an increase in diagnoses and treatments, it is essential to approach tongue ties with a balanced perspective. Not every baby with a tongue tie requires a frenectomy, as many can feed effectively without intervention. However, for those infants who struggle with latching or milk transfer, or cause their mothers significant pain while nursing, a tongue tie can be a genuine barrier to successful breastfeeding. Consulting with a specialist is crucial. These professionals can provide an in-depth assessment of the baby's latch and help determine if a tongue tie is affecting breastfeeding.

How to Achieve a Good Latch

Proper positioning and latching are essential for successful breastfeeding. Here's how to position yourself and your baby for optimal latch:

1. **Find a Comfortable Position** – Make yourself comfortable seated on a bed or sofa, with good back support. Use pillows to support your arms, back and baby if needed. Focus on your comfort first, then bring your baby to your breast, rather than trying to bring your breast to your baby. Bear in mind that there may be times in the early weeks when your baby is cluster feeding for hours at a time.

2. **Position Your Baby** – Hold your baby close to you, with their body and face facing yours and their nose level with

your nipple. Their head should be free to tilt back slightly. Remember, it's essential to bring your baby to your breast, not the other way around. Do not stoop to bring your breasts down to your baby's height – use cushions or a nursing pillow to raise your baby up to the ideal height. Trust me, no-one benefits from you contorting your body into painful positions to nurse. Your neck and back will thank you for not doing so!

3. **Latch Your Baby** – Wait for your baby to open their mouth wide, like a yawn. If they don't do this readily, encourage them to do so by stroking their nose and lips with your nipple. You might even gently squeeze your breast to express a little colostrum, allowing a few droplets to gather on your nipple for your baby to smell. Next, bring your baby to your breast with their chin touching your breast first, then aim their lower lip below your nipple. Once their mouth is wide open, bring them onto your breast, angling your nipple towards the roof of your baby's mouth (this triggers their sucking reflex).

Once latched, your baby's lips should be flanged out like fish lips and the dark area of your nipple should be visible at the top of your breast, but not at the bottom.

To ensure a deep and effective latch, here are some key things to look out for:

- **Sucking and Swallowing:** In the beginning, your baby might suck quickly and shallowly to stimulate your milk flow, but as the milk comes in their sucking should slow and become more rhythmic. You should hear deep sucks followed by the sound of a swallow. If you hear clicking or smacking sounds, this could mean your baby's latch is shallow, and they may be drawing in air.

- **The Rhythm of Feeding:** A deep latch feels steady and consistent. You might feel a slight pull at the start, but the sucking should soon become relaxed and deliberate. If the sucking is inconsistent or if you feel sharp biting pain, it's a sign that the latch may need adjustment.

- **Jaw Movement:** When your baby is latched deeply, their jaw will move rhythmically with each suck. If the jaw doesn't move smoothly or if the sucking feels shallow and fast, your baby may not be latched properly.

- **No Pain:** Once established, breastfeeding should feel comfortable. Some tenderness is normal in the early days or weeks, but excruciating pain and cracked, sore nipples are definitely not something to put up with. Any sharp, stinging or burning pain that lasts beyond a few feeds likely indicates that your baby's latch isn't deep enough, or could even signal an infection like nipple thrush (more on that in Chapter Four, see page 123). In short, if in doubt – get checked out.

- **Nipple Shape After Feeding:** After feeding, your nipple should look round and lengthened like a bullet – and not pinched. If it looks flattened or misshapen, it's a sign that your baby might only be sucking on the tip of your nipple rather than taking in more of the areola. This *may* cause pain and reduce milk transfer.

- **Comfort During and After Feeding:** Breastfeeding should generally feel comfortable once your baby has latched well. If you're feeling persistent pain, it's worth adjusting the latch and seeking help if necessary. That is not to say that some discomfort isn't simply a sign that your nipples are adjusting to doing a job they have never done before. Some tenderness is not necessarily problematic, but if you are in toe-curling pain every time you nurse or pump, do not expect that things will get better by themselves.

If any of these signs sound familiar, seek support as a matter of urgency. Having your baby's latch checked early on can save you a lot of discomfort in the long run. Remember, you don't have to do this alone. With the right guidance, you and your baby will be on your way to a smooth and successful breastfeeding journey.

If anything feels off – whether it's pain, discomfort, concerns about milk supply or your baby's weight gain – reach out for help. Addressing issues early is always easier than waiting until they become more challenging. Whether it's a visit to a local breastfeeding support centre, a consultation with an IBCLC or simply checking in with your midwife or Health Visitor, getting personalised expert support can make all the difference to your breastfeeding experience.

Prioritise Rest and Recovery

How ironic it is that as a new nursing mother adequate rest and sleep are essential, not only for your well-being but also for maintaining your milk supply. Yet rest often feels like an elusive luxury – something just out of reach when your little 'boob monster' keeps you constantly on your toes. But here's the thing – rest isn't just about feeling a little more refreshed or managing the day ahead. It's absolutely critical for your physical and emotional well-being and healing, and it plays a pivotal role in supporting your breastfeeding journey.

I believe one of the biggest contributors to low breastfeeding rates in places like the UK and the US is the pressure new mothers feel to do everything *except* rest during maternity leave. But here's the truth – sleep is when your body's healing process truly kicks in. It's during those moments of rest that your body repairs, regenerates and restores. Your nervous system – already under a lot of stress after birth – needs proper rest to regulate and soothe itself. Without this, it can be challenging to trigger the hormonal balance needed for milk production.

The soothing effects of sleep help you produce prolactin, the hormone responsible for milk production and oxytocin, the hormone that enables your milk to flow. Without enough rest, your nervous system remains on high alert, which can make it harder to trigger the release of these hormones.

Rest is also key for your mental and emotional well-being. The postpartum period can feel overwhelming with so many things on your plate, but your nervous system simply cannot function optimally without it. When you're exhausted, it's much harder to cope with the stresses of new motherhood. It's easy to fall into a cycle of fatigue that feels impossible to break, but the reality is that the more rest you can give yourself, the better your body will respond to breastfeeding and emotional regulation.

Now, I know this is easier said than done. Finding time to rest when you feel like you've got a million things to do or when your baby's feeding schedule is unpredictable can be incredibly difficult. But honestly, one of the biggest lessons I've learned in my own motherhood journey – and what I see echoed by so many families I work with – is that slowing down is absolutely essential. Rest isn't just a luxury; it's the cornerstone of your health and happiness as a new nursing or pumping mother. By consciously deciding to slow down – even in small, bite-sized moments – you're laying the groundwork for a successful, sustainable breastfeeding journey.

Without rest, it's hard to focus on anything else, let alone fully master or 'enjoy' breastfeeding. Rest is not just something to 'catch up on' later – it's crucial to your healing, your milk supply and your overall well-being.

If you're on maternity leave, especially if it's your first baby, I can't emphasise this enough: *rest when your baby is sleeping or not demanding anything from you.* Even if you struggle to sleep, take those moments to relax. Close your eyes, meditate or just breathe slowly and deeply – don't feel the pressure to 'do' anything else like admin or chores. If you're back at work, make your breaks as restful as possible. Whether it's stepping outside for some fresh air or simply sitting in a quiet room for a few minutes, use those moments to recharge rather than running errands. For those of you at home with multiple children, I appreciate how challenging it can be, but you need respite, too. Modern life means that moments don't just happen, you need to build them in.

If you do have older children, carve out small chunks of time each day to unwind and recharge. Whether it's curling up with a good book, switching off as your children listen to an audiobook or letting your older children enjoy some screen time while you sit down for a cup of tea. These small acts of self-care make a world of difference. And it's okay to ask for help – in fact, I would argue that it's vital. Plan to lean on friends and family when you can. Taking care of yourself is not a luxury, but a necessity for both your own well-being and for being able to show up for your children.

Time in nature is another often overlooked tool that I encourage every new mother to embrace. If you have access to a garden or nearby park, even a short walk or a few moments of fresh air can work wonders for your mental clarity and physical recovery. The simple act of stepping outside can help soothe your nervous system, clear your mind and offer a much-needed break from the daily routine. There's something so grounding about nature that reminds us to slow down, breathe deeply and reconnect with ourselves.

Engaging in activities like walking not only provides the benefits of fresh air and natural surroundings but also incorporates bilateral stimulation. This rhythmic, side-to-side movement has been shown to activate both hemispheres of the brain, promoting emotional regulation and reducing stress. Research indicates that such bilateral stimulation can have a calming effect on the nervous system, enhancing your mental well-being.

> ### How to Ask for Help – A Visualisation Exercise
>
> If, like many of my clients – and let's face it, most women in the modern world – you find it difficult to ask for help, let's take a moment together to gently explore that feeling.
>
> Close your eyes and take a few slow, deep breaths. As you inhale, feel your lungs fill from the bottom up, each breath flowing smoothly like the ebb and flow of the tide. Allow each breath to bring a sense of calm into your body. Now, imagine yourself at three or four years old. Picture that sweet smile, the joy you felt when playing, singing and laughing. What were your favourite things to do back then? Who did you love to spend time with? Now imagine that vibrant little girl has grown up and is holding her own baby, needing support just like you do. Doesn't she deserve the same kindness, compassion and help that you would offer? Remember, just like that little girl, you deserve support too – because you are worthy of it just as much as anyone.
>
> Learning to take care of yourself as you take care of your new baby is not about getting it perfect – it's about making wellness matter too. Over time, those little pockets of care add up, and you'll notice a big difference in how you feel, both physically and emotionally. And the best part? It all supports your milk supply, your mental health and your ability to be the loving, present parent you want to be.

Coping with Sleep Deprivation

I could never have anticipated just how exhausting it would be to survive on as little as three or four broken hours of sleep each night for months. Yet, adequate rest is essential for postpartum recovery, hormone regulation and milk production and for some this feels like an unamusing irony. Studies show a clear link between extreme sleep deprivation, chronically heightened stress levels and reduced milk supply. Support from partners, family and friends is invaluable, as it allows you to recuperate, breastfeed on demand and reduce the risk of stress-induced impacts on breastfeeding success – so try to invest in your own rest however you can.

We've all heard the age-old advice, 'Sleep when the baby sleeps.' But how often do we actually follow it? Even if you have older children, I highly recommend that you go to bed as soon as possible after them at nighttime to maximise the hours of sleep that you get. It's all too easy to fall into the trap of using nap time to catch up on laundry, scroll through social media or sneak in that much-needed shower. While the urge to be productive is completely understandable, getting more sleep – *no matter how little* – can make a huge difference to your well-being. The laundry and social media will still be there when your little one wakes, but that opportunity to rest will have passed.

I know, it's not always that simple, right? If you're anything like me, it can feel impossible to fall asleep during the day, even when you're utterly exhausted. Your mind is racing and instead of resting, you end up staring at the ceiling or worrying about the chores piling up and our brains are on high alert for our baby waking. So, if you struggle with this, try something different: sit or lie down and simply close your eyes. You might not drift off immediately, but even just allowing your body to rest and your shoulders to soften will help. If you do happen to fall asleep, even for a few minutes, you'll wake up feeling more refreshed and prepared to face the day than if you had spent the time rushing around, trying to catch up on tasks.

And if sleep continues to evade you, try bringing some calming techniques into your day to soothe your nervous system. A few minutes of deep breathing can work wonders in quieting your mind and restoring your energy. Here are some simple yet powerful yoga breathwork practices to help you recharge:

4-7-8 Breathing

Inhale slowly through your nose for four seconds, hold your breath for seven seconds and exhale slowly through your mouth for eight seconds. This pranayama technique helps activate your parasympathetic nervous system, bringing a sense of calm and helping to reduce anxiety. Even just a few rounds of this can help relax your body and mind.

Nadi Shodhana Pranayama (Alternate Nostril Breathing)

This technique involves inhaling through one nostril and exhaling through the other. You can do this by gently closing one nostril with your thumb, inhaling deeply through the other nostril. Then close that nostril with a finger and exhale through the other nostril. This practice calms your mind, balances your energy and can help you feel more centred when everything around you feels a little chaotic.

Ujjayi Pranayama (Victorious Breath)

Inhale deeply through your nose and exhale slowly (through your nose), while gently constricting your throat, creating a soft, oceanic, 'ha' sound. This technique is great for calming your racing thoughts and relieving mental tension. It's often used in yoga to reduce stress and promote relaxation, which is especially helpful when you're feeling overwhelmed.

Deep, Slow Breaths While Walking

If you find it hard to sit still and breathe, try walking slowly and mindfully. Inhale deeply through your nose for four steps and exhale slowly through your nose for another four steps. Repeat this for a few minutes while walking at a moderate pace. It will help clear your mind and soothe your nervous system, giving you a moment of calm amidst the busyness of new motherhood.

Dirga Pranayama (Three-Part Breath)

This technique involves filling your lungs in three stages. First, inhale deeply into your belly, then your rib cage and finally your chest. Exhale slowly and completely, letting go of any tension in your body. This full, deep breath supports relaxation and helps you reconnect with your body.

These simple breathing exercises can be done in short bursts throughout your day. Even just five minutes of focussed breathing can make a significant difference to how you feel.

Journalling

One way to reconnect with your instincts and figure out what you really need is through journalling. I know, it can feel a little indulgent, especially when you're exhausted, but hear me out: journalling is a powerful tool. It helps you reflect on what you're going through and how you're truly feeling. You might not realise it now, but taking a moment to write can help you sift through the chaos and get a sense of clarity. And this clarity can be exactly what you need to uncover your instincts and begin to feel more grounded in your new milk-centred world.

So, let's take a step back, breathe and make a plan to start with *you*. When it comes to using the prompts throughout this book, you may choose to sit with a pen and paper and write out your thoughts, but journalling doesn't need to be as formal or prescriptive as that. Quite frankly, the opportunities to journal as you might have done pre-motherhood are likely to be few and far between, too. Instead, you might be able to focus on just one or two prompts per day. You can answer them by making notes on your phone, in the margins of this book or even simply contemplating the questions asked. Ready? Here are a few journal prompts to help you make sense of this new, wild and wonderful world you're navigating:

1. **What's been the hardest part of these first few weeks for you?** Is it the physical demands of breastfeeding, the emotional rollercoaster or the sheer exhaustion of trying to balance it all?

2. **When was the last time you felt truly rested or nourished?** (It's normal and okay if the answer is: before you were pregnant.) How can you make sure to prioritise those moments, even in small ways, throughout the day?

3. **What have you been telling yourself about what a 'good mother' should do or be?** What are the unrealistic expectations you're placing on yourself that need to be let go?

4. **What do you need right now – physically, emotionally and mentally?** Take a moment to tune into yourself and acknowledge those needs, no matter how simple they may seem.

5. **What does your ideal breastfeeding experience look like?** What's the reality right now and what small changes could help you feel more comfortable or supported?

By taking a moment to reconnect with yourself through journalling, you can start to make sense of what you really need at this moment. And trust me, this is a huge step towards building a more balanced and compassionate relationship with yourself, which will naturally flow into your new role as a breastfeeding mother. During pregnancy, the neural connections in your brain were pruned in such a way that your mind is primed for love and care. You really have got this – even on the days when it feels like everything's falling apart.

CHAPTER TWO

Finding a Rhythm

This chapter is all about adjusting to life with a newborn. The early weeks of breastfeeding can feel all-encompassing, and you may wonder if you'll ever find a rhythm that feels sustainable. With the blessing of hindsight, I now look back with nostalgia at those first few days and weeks in the knowledge that they stood me in good stead to weather the ever-changing nature of motherhood well beyond the fourth trimester. Between sleep deprivation, feeding sessions that seem to stretch on indefinitely and a body still healing from birth, this chapter is here to help you navigate these early days and weeks and establish a rhythm that works for both you and your baby.

The Early Weeks: Embracing Flexibility

I see you. I hear you. I feel you. The early days of breastfeeding can feel like an endless cycle – exhausting, overwhelming and unrelenting. As one client shared – and many have echoed, 'I wondered what I had done and whether I would ever feel human again?' It's something we're often not prepared for, and it can feel like your energy is being drained in ways you didn't think were possible. But I want you to know that all this feeding has a purpose. Newborns have tiny stomachs and big energy demands, which means they need to nurse frequently – anywhere from 8–12 times in a 24-hour period. Yes, sometimes it is literally constant, but each feed is not just about nourishment for your baby – it's also crucial for establishing your milk supply. Your body is responding to your baby's needs, and with every feed, you're building a steady milk supply that will grow and evolve with your baby.

With the blessing of hindsight, I now look back on those early days with a sense of nostalgia. Yes, they were immeasurably tough, but they also laid the foundation for everything that followed in my motherhood journey. And trust me, a loose sense of rhythm and balance is possible – even amidst the chaos of sleep deprivation, endless feeds and a body still recovering from the physical toll of pregnancy and childbirth.

In my work with mothers around the world, I've seen time and time again that finding that steady rhythm isn't about perfection, but about learning to adapt to the ebbs and flows of your new life. This is often completely at odds with the ways that many of us have lived our lives before parenthood! In this chapter, I'll share the insights and strategies I've used to help many women just like you find that balance – one that works for them, their baby and their family. Together we'll explore how to make this wild, beautiful ride a little bit more manageable and a lot more fulfilling.

I'll never forget the battle I had trying to get out of the house in time for a 10am mother and baby group when my son was just a few weeks old. I had all the best intentions – ready to put on a brave face and embrace the world of new motherhood with a perfect, Instagram-worthy smile. But in reality? I was running on fumes. My son was crying, I was flustered under my makeup and the clock seemed to tick faster with every minute that passed. Looking back, I can see clearly that the real issue wasn't the rush to make it to that group, but my own perception of what I should be doing day-to-day. I'd been so focussed on what other mothers were posting – picture-perfect moments of motherhood that made everything seem effortless – that I forgot to take care of the basics. I skipped meals, barely slept and on the rare occasions that my son fell asleep, I rushed around like a headless chicken trying to tidy up, cook and keep up appearances. I wish I could go back and simply give myself a big hug.

But let's stop for a moment and think about *you* and your needs. It's so easy to forget: your needs matter just as much as your precious newborn's. In those early days, the fourth trimester can be a blur of feeding, changing, soothing and trying to make everything look perfect. It's easy to lose track of your own well-being when everything seems so urgent and overwhelming. Your baby's needs are at the forefront and your own are put on the back burner. For many of us too, we do not have extended family lining up to drop off food parcels and take care of us as we heal. So, here's a gentle reminder: you need to start with yourself *first*. We've touched on this in Chapter One, but it bears repeating – recognising your own needs can be one of the hardest things to do in the haze of new motherhood. It might feel a little too simple or even obvious to say, but it's essential to pause and check in with yourself. As discussed in Chapter One, journalling is a beautiful and impactful way to do this.

Feeding in the First Six Weeks

As the first week goes on, you'll notice that your baby will need to feed regularly – more often than you might expect. I have lost count of the number of mothers I have spoken to who are shocked that their newborn babies sometimes nurse for hours at a time (and who express disbelief that this can be normal!). I think I have stressed enough now how frequent feeds in those early days are crucial for helping your body establish a full milk supply. In fact, the most significant increase in your baby's milk intake usually happens during the first three weeks. Now, I know it might feel like your baby is always on the breast, but this really is a good thing! By nursing whenever your baby shows hunger cues, your milk supply will naturally adjust to meet their growing needs, supporting their healthy growth and development.

Crying is usually the last sign of hunger, so if your baby's already crying, it can be a little harder to settle them and latch. It's all about catching those earlier signs (see below), so you can respond promptly and avoid reaching the point where your baby is feeling frustrated or too upset to latch easily. In short, watch your baby, not just the clock, and within no time you will be able to recognise when your little one needs a feed.

Frequent nursing, also known as cluster feeding, is vital for establishing your milk supply in those early days, weeks and months. It also fosters a lovely, comforting connection between you and your baby. The more you nurse, the more your milk supply will increase to keep up with your baby's demands – so trust your body, trust your baby and lean into the evolving rhythm of it all.

So, what do hunger cues look like? Here are some key signs to watch for:

1. **Rooting:** Your baby turns their head towards your breast, opening their mouth and making sucking motions, often when their cheek is gently stroked.

2. **Sucking on their hands or fingers:** Babies often bring their hands to their mouth when they're hungry.

3. **Lip Smacking:** If your baby's lips are smacking or they're making sucking noises, it's a good indication that they're ready to feed.

4. **Fussiness or Whining:** They may start to get fussy, making noises or appearing unsettled as they start to feel hungry.

5. **Increased alertness or rooting around:** Your baby might start rooting around on your chest, searching for your nipple.

6. **Rapid eye movements:** Your baby might exhibit quicker eye movements or look for your breast with wide eyes, signalling they're hungry.

What's Normal?

Sometimes babies seem to be constantly wanting to be on the boob, so you may wonder whether your baby truly needs another feed. This uncertainty can be heightened by well-meaning but unhelpful unsolicited advice from friends and family, leaving you feeling overwhelmed with self-doubt. Rest assured that as long as your baby is well-hydrated (as shown by their nappy output), gaining weight at the expected rate and nursing feels comfortable and pain-free, there is no reason to worry if they want to nurse frequently or for long periods. On the contrary, nursing on demand is absolutely vital for establishing and maintaining a healthy milk supply.

After the first week, your baby will start to take in more milk at each feed. On average, they'll begin taking in about 425–710ml (15–25oz) of milk a day. By the time they're around 2–3 weeks old, that's typically around 57–85ml (2–3oz) per feed. If your baby is exclusively breastfed, there really is no way to actively track how much milk they are drinking at each feed – and there is no need to, either. I share these numbers as a point of reference only. You may find them helpful *if* you are bottle feeding alongside nursing. After three weeks, you might notice that the frequency of feeds starts to settle a little bit, although the amount of milk your baby needs continues to grow as they get bigger. By the end of the first month, many babies are consuming between 710ml and 994ml (25oz and 35oz) of milk a day, though individual needs can vary quite a lot. Some babies may need less, others more – and guess what? Both are completely normal!

Now, I know that thinking about millilitres when breastfeeding can be a bit baffling. In fact, if you're anything like I was in the early days, it might make you feel like you're chasing a number you can't possibly catch. I really want to emphasise that breastfeeding isn't about measuring milk every time you nurse. It's about nursing on demand, around the clock, *for the rest of your life* (I'm joking!).

And I totally understand if you're feeling overwhelmed at the thought of counting all those millilitres – unless you're pumping or formula feeding, in which case, you're probably already juggling those numbers.

Here is an outline of roughly how many millilitres your baby is likely to need during the fourth trimester within a 24-hour period:

Your Baby's Age	Your Baby's Weight	Number of Feeds	Total No. of ml/oz in 24 Hours
3 Days	-	8–12	15–30ml (0.5–1oz) per feed, total 90–120ml (3–4oz)
1 Week	-	8–12	45–60ml (1.5–2oz) per feed, total 360–480ml (12–16 oz)
2 Weeks	-	8–12	60–90 ml (2–3oz) per feed, total 480–720ml (16–24oz)
1 Month	10–12lbs (4.5–5.4kg)	8–12	90–120ml (3–4oz) per feed, total 720–960ml (24–32oz)
6 Weeks	12lbs (5.4kg)	8–10	120ml (4oz) per feed, total 720–900ml (24–30oz)
3 Months	14–15lbs (6.4–6.8kg)	7–9	120–150ml (4–5oz) per feed, total 750–900ml (25–30oz)

As you may have been told, it can be helpful to keep in mind that your newborn needs to nurse at least every three hours until they are around two weeks old or they have regained their birth weight. You'll start to get into the rhythm of things and before long you'll find that breastfeeding feels more natural and less about trying to hit a target.

App or No App?

There are a multitude of different apps available for tracking your baby's every waking and sleeping move. I completely understand why they exist and why some mothers find them helpful. However, I would err on the side of caution before you consider downloading one. This is particularly true if you – like me and many of my clients – have perfectionist tendencies.

Similarly, if you feel anxious about your baby's food intake, regular alerts from various apps may contribute to your anxiety levels rather than helping you feel more in control. The perhaps jarring truth is that we cannot control our babies any more than we can control any of the people we love! Contrary to outdated, behaviourist beliefs about babies and children, they are all as unique as every one of us. As such, it is normal for it to take time to get to know your baby – whether you have the assistance of an app or not.

Importantly, and however exhausting, many babies nurse most frequently between 9pm and 3am in the first few months, taking in up to 20 per cent of their total daily calories at night. Honestly, when you are recovering from pregnancy and labour, it can feel like pure torture to be kept awake during the hours when you are sleepiest. One client recalled how she had briefly fantasised about throwing her tiny baby out of the window after she woke for the millionth time that night, as she thought to herself, 'At least then I could get some sleep.'

It's vital to acknowledge that these moments of pure exhaustion are real, and they don't make you a bad mother. You are not alone in feeling like this, and it doesn't mean you aren't doing your best. The early days of motherhood can feel overwhelming, and it's okay to admit when things feel too much.

Intrusive Thoughts – What to Watch For

Intrusive thoughts are an all-too-common experience for many new parents, particularly in those early days of exhaustion. These are sudden, unwanted and often disturbing thoughts that pop into your mind without warning. It can be anything from fearing harm might come to your baby to ideas of running away from the responsibility of parenting. While these thoughts are upsetting, it's important to remember that *they do not define you* and *do not mean you will act on them.*

However, if these intrusive thoughts become more frequent, intense or are accompanied by feelings of extreme anxiety, hopelessness or disconnection, they can be indicative of a more serious condition such as postpartum psychosis. This is a rare but critical mental health concern that requires immediate attention.

Signs you should Seek Help:

- Persistent overwhelming thoughts that are difficult to control.
- Feelings of detachment from reality, such as not recognising the importance of your thoughts.

- Extreme fear of harming yourself or your baby or having visions of violence.
- Intense mood swings, paranoia or an inability to feel connected to your baby.

If you or someone you know is experiencing these symptoms, it's crucial to seek help immediately. Postpartum psychosis can be treated with professional intervention, and the sooner you reach out, the better the outcome.

The reality is that from an anthropological perspective, we were never meant to parent in isolation and yet, that is how most of us live. The impact upon our collective mental health as mothers is undeniably momentous and so we all need to give ourselves some grace. If these thoughts become more frequent or if you find yourself feeling persistently down, anxious or disconnected, please ask for help. Seeking support for your mental health is a sign of strength and in time it will set an excellent precedent for your child. Whether it's talking to a trusted friend, a health visitor or a professional, support is available and it can make all the difference in navigating these challenging moments. You will get through this – one moment at a time. Head to the resources section of this book for more information about where to find professional postpartum mental health support (see page 305).

Night-time Feeding

Whilst overnight feeding can be incredibly challenging, it plays an essential role in ensuring adequate milk intake and supporting milk supply during these early months. To make nighttime feedings more manageable, try creating a comfortable setup near your bed. Keeping a low light, your water bottle and a few snacks nearby can make night feedings easier. These small changes also allow you to keep the room calm and quiet, helping both you and your baby to settle back to sleep more easily. You may find that practising safe co-sleeping (sharing a bed or other surface with your baby) makes night feeding less disruptive; others prefer using a bassinet close to the bed. The Lullaby Trust offers the most up-to-date information and research on safe cosleeping. I discuss night feeding in more depth on page 59.

Finding What Works for You and Your Baby's Safety and Comfort

To help you find a rhythm that works for both you and your baby at night, consider implementing a plan that allows you to share the load with a partner or family support. This can provide much-needed relief, help you recharge and ultimately set the stage for a better day ahead. Here are some practical ways to make night-time care more manageable:

1. **Create a Shifting Sleep Schedule:** If you have a partner or support, try setting up a shift system. One parent could go to bed early, around 8pm, to get a solid stretch of rest before the night shift begins. The other parent could sleep from 1am to 6am, after the first shift. This way, both parents get a decent block of uninterrupted sleep, allowing for much-needed recovery.

2. **Take Turns with Feeding:** If you're breastfeeding or combi-feeding, this approach can also work well if you're pumping breast milk. One parent can give a bottle of pumped milk during the night feedings, allowing the other parent to get a bit of extra rest. Bear in mind if you do this, you will still need to wake up to pump to make

up for the feed that you missed overnight in order to maintain your milk supply.

3. **Nappy Changes and Settling Baby:** Remember, it's not just about feeding. Nappy changes and soothing the baby back to sleep can interrupt your sleep just as much. Make sure to share these responsibilities so that one parent isn't doing all the work while the other is trying to sleep. If one person handles the feed, the other could focus on soothing the baby back to sleep. This can help you get a few more moments of precious sleep.

4. **Support with Household Tasks:** Although you may find yourself home alone for much of the time during maternity leave, this doesn't mean you should shoulder all the household responsibilities yourself. Maternity leave is a time for you to rest and recover from pregnancy and childbirth – not a time to spend every waking hour keeping your home in perfect order. If you can afford it, consider hiring a cleaner once a week, subscribing to a meal delivery service or sending your laundry out to be done. Do this guilt-free, knowing that you deserve all the support you can get. If this is beyond your budget, ask friends or family to take turns helping with a meal train or a cleaning rota. If you feel uncomfortable asking them directly, ask someone you trust to reach out on your behalf. And remember, if they ever need help in the future, you can always return the favour. Our 'villages' may look different these days, but that gives us the opportunity to set a new, supportive precedent for future generations.

5. **Recharging for the Day Ahead:** Taking time for yourself, even if it's just a few hours of uninterrupted sleep, is essential for maintaining your physical and emotional

well-being. It can help you feel more capable and supported when you're back on duty the next day. Prioritising your own rest is not selfish – it's necessary to be the best parent you can be.

Ultimately, there's no 'one size fits all' approach to parenting, and it's about finding what works best for you and your family. But by incorporating shifts, sharing responsibilities and using whatever support you have effectively, you really can ease the load and create a more balanced routine for both yourself and your baby.

How to Give Yourself Grace as a No-sleep Nursing Mama

As a new nursing mum, you are likely exhausted, overwhelmed and still trying to figure out how to meet your baby's needs while taking care of yourself. In the middle of the sleepless nights and the endless feeds, it can be hard to give yourself grace. You may feel like you should be able to do it all – nurse on demand, keep the house running, be fully present with your baby – and still manage to feel *somewhat* like yourself. This is the story that I hear from my clients on a daily basis. But here's the truth: you *are* doing enough. Just by being there for your baby, just by holding space for their needs, you are more than enough.

Let's take a moment to breathe and allow ourselves to drop the heavy, unrealistic expectations. Close your eyes if you can, and take a deep breath in. Feel your body expand with air, filling you with calm. Take a few deep breaths in and out, filling your lungs from bottom to top. Now exhale and imagine that all the pressure you've been carrying melts away with your breath. Let it go.

Now, repeat after me, 'I don't have to have to have it all together, all of the time. Just like my baby, I am just as deserving of love and kindness when I am struggling as when I am thriving.'

I know you might feel like your to-do list is never-ending and that there's always more you could be doing, but grace is about recognising that there is no perfect way to navigate new motherhood. If you're struggling to sleep, to nourish yourself, to find time for yourself, it's okay. You don't need to do it all right now. The myth that you do is a vastly unjust one in modern motherhood. The world will still be there when you're ready and so will your baby. In the meantime – and at all times – you deserve nothing but kindness from yourself.

I encourage you to let go of striving for perfection and embrace the beautiful, fleeting messiness of this phase. How? Self-compassion isn't about getting everything done; it's about giving yourself permission to *not* do everything. It's about allowing yourself to rest, to slow down and to care for yourself – even when the to-do list feels endless. One way to do this is by focussing on *glimmers*, the opposite of triggers. Small, uplifting moments or actions throughout the day that give you hope and joy. Pay attention to them: did your newborn flash you their first little smile (even if it was just wind!)? Did you manage to take a shower today? Woohoo! Or perhaps you and your baby are fed, watered and rested – what a victory in the whirlwind of the fourth trimester! Every day, choose just one small thing you're proud of and let that small but mighty win be enough for today.

Global Inspiration

Whilst I hope this is not true for you, in my experience and in the experience of many of the mums I work with, a nursing mother's role is often grossly undervalued. In a society where productivity is king, this is in stark contrast to the deliberately slow and healing pace that new mothers need. Many cultures around the world have long-standing postpartum practices where new mothers are cared for deeply, surrounded by their families and communities for weeks, sometimes even months after childbirth.

For example, in China the postpartum period is called *zuò yuè zi*, which translates to 'doing the month'. During this time, new mothers are often confined to the house and receive daily massages (yes please!), to help with recovery and to boost milk production. In India, the postpartum period is known as *jaapa* (sometimes spelt *japa*), a 40-day confinement period where new mothers are cared for by family members and members of the community who support them with housework, cooking and baby care, allowing them to focus on resting and bonding with their baby.

Similarly, in Japan, *osouji* refers to a 100-day confinement period where new mothers are cared for by family members and their primary responsibility is to rest and recover, while their family takes care of daily tasks. Meanwhile in South Korea, the postpartum period is called *sanhujori*, a 21-day confinement period where new mothers avoid going outside or receiving guests, ensuring they can fully rest and heal in the early days after birth.

Modern life in the traditional West has robbed many modern mothers of this *vital* care and support. The demands of work and social expectations have made it difficult for new mothers to receive the nurturing and rest they desperately need during the postpartum period. And so – as if we aren't already doing enough – we must reimagine this care for ourselves. We must establish our own postnatal rituals, advocate for the support we deserve and make space for the rest and healing that we need. Whether that means seeking help from family and friends, outsourcing household tasks or simply giving ourselves permission to rest without guilt, potentially in a messy home.

I appreciate that this is not easy to do, especially when you are so wholly consumed by new motherhood – so let's do it together. In this chapter I draw upon the collective wisdom of so many of the wonderful mothers I have worked with to help you carve out postpartum boundaries that work for you.

Journal Prompts

Here is a selection of journal prompts designed to help you practise self-compassion, reflect on your journey and embrace your experience with grace during the postpartum period:

1. **I am so proud of myself for...**
   Celebrate your victories, big and small, no matter how trivial they may have seemed before you were a parent. Reflect on moments where you took care of yourself, your baby or how you made it through a difficult day.

2. **One of the hardest things I did today was...**
   This is about acknowledging your struggles. It's important to recognise the challenges that you overcome, as they're part of your growth. So, what made today tough and how did you navigate it?

3. **My body is amazing because...**
   Shift your focus to your body's incredible strength and resilience. How has it evolved in the last few weeks or months? Where does it need more care and attention?

4. **I am in awe of how my baby...**
   Write down a moment today that filled you with wonder. Whether it's a smile, a coo or a new milestone, let yourself soak in the beauty of your baby's growth.

5. **My mind is amazing because ...**
   Take a moment to recognise your mind's ever-changing power and adaptability. Think about just how much you have grown since your baby was born.

6. **Being pregnant was hard, but the thing that makes this season hard is ...**
   Reflect on the challenges that come with this postpartum period. How do they compare to pregnancy? Acknowledge the difficulties while also recognising your strength.

7. **Looking back on pregnancy, I realise now that ...**
   Take a moment to reflect on what you've learned since becoming a mother. How has your perspective shifted in these early weeks and months?

8. **The thing I enjoy most about caring for my baby right now is ...**
   It's almost impossible not to get caught up in the exhaustion, but take a moment to focus on what brings you joy. What part of this journey is most fulfilling for you?

9. **The hardest part about being a new parent is ...**
   It's important to acknowledge the tough moments. Where do you struggle? Be gentle with yourself here.

10. **Today I am grateful for ...**
    Gratitude can be a powerful tool for mental well-being. Find five things in your day – no matter how small – to feel thankful for.

11. **Being a mother means ...**
    Reflect on what motherhood is to you. What has it taught you about yourself? How has it already shaped your sense of identity? How can you *embrace* those changes rather than resisting them?

12. **My favourite way to care for myself these days is ...**
    What achievable self-care rituals make a difference in your life right now? Whether it's a quiet cup of tea or five minutes of deep breathing, focus on how you can nurture yourself.

13. **The five things I want to remember from this postpartum period are ...**
    Take a moment to imagine what you want to carry forward with you. What are the lessons, feelings or moments you want to hold onto?

14. **I feel loved best during this postpartum period when ...**
    Reflect on the ways you feel supported. Is it a hug from a loved one? A thoughtful gesture from a friend? Remember that love comes in many forms. Carry that love with you throughout your days and especially nights.

15. **Motherhood could best be described as ...**
    If you could sum up motherhood in a word or phrase, what would it be? What feelings or emotions come up when you think about this new chapter?

By journalling on these prompts, you'll open yourself up to understanding your emotions and the nuances of your postpartum experience. Most importantly, you'll give yourself permission to embrace the grace and compassion you truly deserve.

How Often Should I Breastfeed My Baby?

Each baby is unique and so are we as mothers. Remember those incredible milk-making cells called lactocytes we discussed in Chapter One? Well, each of us has a unique number of them. Some mothers have larger storage capacities than others, which means their babies might get more milk per feed and potentially go longer between feeds. And just to clear up a common misconception – this has nothing to do with breast size! That's right, the size of your breasts does not correlate with the amount of milk they can hold at any given time.

Exclusively breastfed babies typically nurse around eight times a day, but anywhere from 8–12 times is completely normal. Some babies feed quickly and efficiently, while others prefer to linger, enjoying a longer, more leisurely feed. Depending on your situation, personality and circumstances, you might find that shorter, more frequent feeding sessions feel great to you, breaking up long stretches of time. Alternatively, you may prefer prolonged feedings, which give you a chance to catch up on Netflix, listen to an audiobook or even steal a quiet moment to rest your eyes.

As your baby becomes more adept at nursing and your milk supply adjusts to meet their needs, feeding frequency may reduce slightly. However, the best guidance is to let your baby take the lead. The clock is not a measure of hunger – your baby's cues are. It is also worth remembering that breastfeeding offers nutrition, hydration and closeness, all of which are essential to your baby's well-being. Sometimes your baby may need food, other times a drink, and all the time, they need the comfort and security of being close to you. There is not necessarily any way to know why they may want to nurse at any time, which is another reason why nursing on demand is so crucial.

Many new mothers feel pressured to identify whether or not their babies are 'just' nursing for comfort, as if that need is less valid than any other. Please be assured, right here and right now, that whether you are a newborn baby or an elderly person, love and comfort are as vital for your well-being as food and water.

It has been said that when a baby is nursing, they are not simply having a meal but are participating in a 'dynamic, bidirectional biological dialogue' where physical, biochemical, hormonal and emotional exchanges are constantly taking place. In essence, you are building a bond with your baby, establishing a foundation for attachment, immunity, cognitive development and so much more – all through this extraordinary act of breastfeeding.

The Role of Night Feeding

Night feeding is an essential part of breastfeeding, supporting milk supply and helping your baby meet their nutritional needs, especially in the early weeks. Babies naturally wake during the night and whether they are breastfed or formula-fed, it's common for them to feed at night. Studies involving over 700 babies aged 6–12 months indicate that 80 per cent woke at least once during the night, regardless of whether they were breast- or bottle-fed. Interestingly, breastfeeding mothers and their partners tend to get around 45 minutes more sleep per night than those who formula-feed. This benefit comes from the unique effects of breastfeeding, which releases relaxing hormones like oxytocin and prolactin, promoting restful, deeper sleep for both mother and baby.

Facts like these can be difficult to accept when everyone at your local baby group claims their five-month-old has been sleeping through the night for weeks. I have vivid memories of feeling like a complete failure as a mother for not somehow being able to 'train' my son to sleep overnight. I wish I had known then that by nursing my boy on demand, I was supporting the establishment of a healthy sleep routine grounded in love and security. So, remember, if you're waking up for night feeds, you're not alone – most parents are right there with you, navigating the ups and downs of night-time parenting. Trust that responding to your baby's needs at night is building a foundation of comfort, trust and well-being that will benefit you both in ways that go far beyond sleep.

Babies' Night-waking Patterns

It's not simply what babies are fed that determines whether they wake at night but rather their developmental stage and temperament. Babies naturally wake more frequently than adults as part of their growth and development. Interestingly, feeding your baby formula or introducing solid foods does not necessarily reduce night waking. In some cases, doing so actually increases night wakes due to digestive discomfort from new foods. Your baby's night waking and feeding patterns gradually shift over time, and eventually their need for night-time feeds will reduce.

Night waking also plays a protective role. Research into Sudden Infant Death Syndrome (SIDS) suggests that babies who wake more frequently may have some protection, as this level of alertness can help prevent SIDS. An analysis of 288 studies on SIDS and breastfeeding confirmed that breastfeeding lowers the risk of SIDS, with exclusive breastfeeding providing even stronger protection.

If you are drowning in the trenches of sleep deprivation right now, I see you, mama. Knowing that night waking has a protective effect on your baby doesn't make coping with being perpetually exhausted any easier. I was that mum – shocked and mortified to hear that no one else's baby was waking up hourly to nurse overnight. I felt like such a failure. What was I doing wrong? Why was everyone else's baby a better sleeper than mine?

If you have asked yourself these same questions, I want to share Hannah's story with you. She reached out to me when her baby, Elodie, was nine months old. She was desperate for help with balancing self-care alongside nursing her daughter. Since the day Elodie was born, she had woken up every 45–60 minutes overnight and would only go back to sleep at the breast. Hannah had worked with her Health Visitor and GP to rule out issues like allergies, sleep apnoea or oral ties, and as far as they could tell, there were no underlying conditions causing Elodie's wakefulness. Hannah was broken, both physically and mentally, and simply didn't know what to do. She was also under constant criticism from friends and family for continuing to nurse her baby girl on demand. Yet despite the exhaustion, Hannah loved breastfeeding because it felt like the only part of motherhood that she was doing right.

From our first consultation together, I suspected that a significant part of the issue was the vicious cycle of Hannah's stress and anxiety levels, which were triggering her nervous system to essentially tell her body and mind that it was not safe to rest. As a bundle of intuition, I suspected that Elodie might be sensing all of this from her mother and as a result, her nervous system was telling her that she needed to check in with her mum between every single sleep cycle. Over the course of three months, we worked together to maximise the rest that Hannah was getting, drawing upon her support network to give her some much-needed me-time, and most importantly, equipping her with skills for self-regulation that would see her through the ever-changing rollercoaster of new parenthood. I heard from Hannah a few months later and by 18 months old, Elodie was sleeping three- or four-hour stretches overnight.

If, like me, you know exactly how Hannah was feeling, you are not alone and I want to reassure you that this particular season of motherhood won't last until your child goes to college – honest. No child nurses forever and each one learns to fall asleep independently in their own time. Until then, know that each wakeful moment is part of your child's healthy development – and by responding to them, you're not only meeting their needs but also supporting their safety and well-being. Trust the process and be gentle with yourself during these early stages, knowing that you're fostering the globally recognised, strongest possible foundation for your baby's growth.

Understanding Feeding Patterns and Cluster Feeding

Babies, especially newborns, tend to follow feeding patterns that vary throughout the day and night. You may notice that your baby cluster feeds – nursing frequently in short intervals during certain parts of the day, typically in the late afternoon or evening. While this can be exhausting, cluster feeding is perfectly normal and signals your baby's desire for extra nourishment and closeness. This pattern also supports your milk supply as it adjusts to meet your baby's growing demands.

During these intense feeding periods, try to settle into a comfortable spot, prepare some water and snacks nearby and consider it an opportunity to rest or watch something you enjoy. Remember, cluster feeding is temporary.

Creating a Feeding Log: When Routine Meets Flexibility

While a rigid schedule may be unrealistic – because our babies, like us, are not robots – some parents find comfort in using a feeding log to help identify patterns. Tracking when your baby feeds, for how long and on which breast can help you anticipate feeding times and give you a sense of when you might get a break. This can also offer a little extra reassurance, especially when you're wondering if your baby's feeding habits are 'normal'. Many apps are available to help track feedings, nappies and sleep, or you may use your phone Notes or simply keep a notepad nearby. The key is remembering that this is a tool to support you, *not* a set of rigid rules to follow. For those who like a bit more structure, a loose routine based on your baby's cues can help establish a rhythm that feels natural. Over time, you'll likely notice a predictable flow of feeding, awake time and naps. In general, keeping feeding sessions relaxed, flexible and responsive to your baby's needs will create a natural rhythm, even if it looks different day by day.

If you find yourself feeling anxious or overwhelmed by tracking feeds, take a deep breath and give yourself permission to stop. The truth is, you don't have to track every detail to be a great parent. What matters most is that you are nourishing your baby with love and care, and that you are meeting their needs in the way that feels best for you both. And if you ever find yourself feeling like tracking is adding more pressure, take a step back. You are not failing if you choose to focus on being present with your baby, rather than zoning in on numbers or charts. Trust yourself – again, this journey isn't about perfection, it's about progress. Even when it doesn't feel that way, you are growing and learning every day alongside your precious baby.

By the time my son was around four months old, I was tracking his weight obsessively, linking how much he grew (or didn't grow) to my self-worth. If you find yourself falling into this same trap of measuring, comparing and worrying about how everything 'should' look, please take a deep breath. Your worth is not tied to the number on the scale or the specific amount of milk your baby drinks. Again, *your worth is not tied to the number on the scale or the specific amount of milk your baby drinks.* You are doing an incredible job by showing up each and every day, nurturing your baby with love and care and providing them with the comfort they need. If you feel like the pressure of tracking your baby's feeds is weighing you down, remember that the most important thing is that you are present for your baby, doing your best in each moment.

> ### Postpartum Anxiety
>
> Postpartum anxiety can sometimes creep in when we feel like we're not doing enough, or when we get caught up in measuring everything. It can be overwhelming, especially when you feel like your efforts aren't yielding the 'right' results. Keep an eye out for these signs of anxiety:
>
> - You feel overwhelmed by small tasks or feel like you're constantly falling short.
>
> - Your mind races with worries, often about things outside of your control, like your baby's growth or how much milk you're producing.
>
> - You find it difficult to focus on the present moment, constantly replaying your actions or decisions in your head.
>
> - You have physical symptoms like a racing heart, trouble sleeping or a constant sense of tension or unease.

If any of this resonates with you, please seek help from your Health Visitor or family doctor. None of us were ever meant to mother alone and all of us need support sometimes.

Seeking the help that you need is a sign of strength and resilience that will serve you way beyond your breastfeeding journey.

Understanding Your Own Rhythms

Alongside finding a rhythm for feeding, it's important to listen to *your* body and find moments to meet your own needs. Breastfeeding is incredibly demanding, both physically and emotionally. As you nurse, your body is expending energy to produce milk, while releasing hormones like oxytocin that promote relaxation and bonding. However, this relaxation hormone can also lead to sudden feelings of drowsiness or hunger, especially when you're low on sleep or energy.

To help stay energised, keep easy-to-reach snacks and water bottles in your main feeding areas and try to prioritise rest when possible. Even short naps can make a significant difference. If naps feel impossible, consider simply resting beside your baby or enjoying a few moments of quiet. Tuning in to your body's cues and finding small ways to recharge will help you sustain your energy for the days ahead.

Introducing Your Baby to Day and Night Patterns

Babies are born without an established circadian rhythm, meaning they don't initially recognise the difference between day and night. This can make night-time feeds particularly challenging, as they simply do not understand why it's time to sleep. However, there are intuitive, gentle ways you can help your baby begin to understand day and night patterns. During the day, keep feeds and activities stimulating – expose your baby to natural light, engage in regular conversations or noises and provide opportunities for active interaction. These cues help your baby understand that daytime is for wakefulness and activity. On the other hand, during night feeds, try to keep things calm and peaceful. Dim the lights, speak quietly and keep the atmosphere soothing, signalling to your baby that it's time for rest and sleep. Over time, your baby will begin to associate dark and quiet with night-time rest.

Your breast milk also plays a significant role in helping establish these patterns. As we touched upon earlier in the book, the hormonal fluctuations in your milk throughout the day naturally support the development of your baby's circadian rhythm. During the daytime, your breast milk contains higher levels of stimulating hormones like cortisol, which can help keep your baby alert and engaged. In contrast, during the evening and night, your milk has increased levels of melatonin – the hormone that promotes sleep and relaxation. Melatonin not only helps your baby feel more sleepy but also aids in the development of their own internal clock.

This is particularly important if you express or pump milk for your baby to be fed when you are apart. This is why it is important to label your expressed milk as 'day milk' or 'night milk' and to give it to your baby at the corresponding times. This will help reinforce these natural hormonal cues, further supporting the establishment of healthy sleep routines. Over time, most babies will naturally start sleeping for longer stretches at night, though this varies *widely* from one little one to another.

If your baby continues to wake frequently throughout the night, like the numerous examples in this book, it might simply be a normal part of their development. However, there are times when persistent wakefulness could be a sign of something else, such as discomfort, hunger or an underlying issue like reflux or allergies. If you have concerns, it's always a good idea to consult with a healthcare professional who can provide guidance tailored to your baby's needs.

Finding a Rhythm in Breastfeeding: Embracing Adaptability

Finding a rhythm in breastfeeding is ultimately about embracing adaptability. When I was a teacher I thrived on structure. My days were meticulously planned and I believed that a rigid and predictable schedule was the key to being a successful mother. I thought that if I could simply implement a timetable for everything – feeding, naps, playtime – everything would fall into place. Perhaps, like me, you also thought that the skills you honed at work would make motherhood feel just as structured and controlled. But as anyone who's been through the whirlwind of new motherhood can tell you, babies have their own ideas about what works best. And, of course, babies don't come with a schedule.

As a new mother, I struggled to embrace the beautiful chaos that is the fourth trimester and beyond. My Type-A personality was firmly rooted in 'shoulds'. I *should* be able to get my baby to sleep by a certain hour. I *should* be able to breastfeed for a set amount of time and be done. I *should* have a predictable routine that worked. I quickly realised, however, that my need for order and predictability didn't mesh with the messy, unpredictable reality of caring for a newborn.

Babies grow quickly and just as you settle into one routine, a developmental leap, a growth spurt or a teething phase will throw everything off. You might find that your little one, who used to feed every three hours, now wants to nurse every hour during a cluster feeding session. Or perhaps, just when you think you've figured out a solid sleep schedule, your baby decides that they now prefer a different rhythm. And that's okay. Because a rhythm doesn't mean a strict schedule – it means a flow that allows for change, a flow that bends and adapts to the needs of your baby, to the needs of you both.

As one of your baby's primary caregivers, or perhaps their sole caregiver, there is no person on this planet better equipped to care for them than you. You know your baby better than anyone else – those little sounds, those subtle cues, the way they snuggle in when they're full, or the way they wriggle when they're uncomfortable. Trust that you and your baby are learning together. Every adjustment you make, each moment of frustration or joy is part of building that deep, resilient bond that will carry you both through this journey.

Struggling to trust yourself? You're not alone. Trust takes time, especially when the world around us can be full of advice and expectations that feel overwhelming. But trust me, mama, you've got this. To help find your own rhythm, ask yourself these questions, perhaps as you are nursing or pumping for your baby:

- **What does my baby need from me right now?** Is it food, comfort or my presence? Don't worry if you don't know the answer straight away! This will get easier with time and practice.

- **How do I feel in this moment?** Do I feel frustrated, calm, exhausted or content? Honour that feeling rather than fighting against it.

- **What would make this moment easier?** Do I need more support, a break or a few minutes of peace?

- **What have I learned today, about myself and my baby?** Each day really is a new lesson if you allow it to be. Please don't worry if you simply don't have the capacity for learning today, tomorrow is a new day and sometimes the lesson is simply knowing and honouring our limits.

- **What small joy can I take from today?** Even if it's just a quiet cuddle or a moment when your baby smiled at you, actively give yourself permission to cherish it.

Embracing Adaptability through Yoga and Mindfulness

Finding a rhythm is ultimately about embracing adaptability – something I've come to understand deeply through my background as a yoga and meditation teacher. Finding a sense of peace and tuning into your instincts as a new mother is not about forcing things into place or adhering to rigid expectations. Instead, it's about flowing with what *is*, adjusting as we go and offering ourselves the same compassion we would offer our loved ones.

In yoga, we practise Yama – moral disciplines – and one of the first teachings is non-violence (Ahimsa), which I believe applies to how we treat ourselves as mothers. Being gentle with your body and offering compassion to yourself, especially during the physical and emotional demands of breastfeeding, is vital. When I let go of my 'shoulds' and accepted the messiness of motherhood, I began to soften into what I would previously have perceived as complete bedlam! Yes, babies, toddlers and young children wake up multiple times a night. Yes, they may change their sleeping and feeding patterns day to day. And yes, you might feel like you're not 'getting it right', but being concerned about getting everything 'right' is a testament to the fact that you are giving your all to this all-consuming, ever-changing role.

As mothers, we often experience physical strain, especially when breastfeeding for long periods. The posture required to hold and nurse your baby can create tension in the back, shoulders and arms. This is where yoga's Asana (postures) come in. Simple yoga stretches can release tension and help alleviate these aches. These stretches not only ease muscle tightness but also encourage relaxation and mindfulness during the caregiving process.

Before beginning any exercise routine, it's important to ensure that your body is ready for gentle movements, especially in the postpartum period. Please consult with your family doctor or healthcare provider to confirm that it's appropriate for you to resume gentle exercises such as yoga.

For instance, in the **Cat-Cow Stretch** (*Marjaryasana-Bitilasana*), follow these steps:

1. Start on your hands and knees in a tabletop position.

2. Keeping your arms straight, as you inhale, arch your back and let your chest open, allowing your belly to drop towards the floor. This is the 'Cow' pose.

3. On your exhale, push through your arms and round your spine upwards towards the ceiling, tucking your chin towards your chest, and drawing your belly button towards your spine for the 'Cat' pose.

4. Flow between these two postures for several breaths, allowing your spine to gently stretch and release tension with each movement.

Another great pose is the **Seated Forward Bend** (*Paschimottanasana*). Here's how to do it:

1. Sit on the floor with your legs extended straight in front of you.

2. Inhale as you lengthen your spine, and as you exhale, gently hinge forward at the hips, reaching for your thighs, shins or feet depending on your flexibility. Keep your chest open until you reach your 'edge' and then allow your back to round as you do so.

3. Hold this posture as you breathe deeply into the space that you are creating along your spine and hamstrings.

4. This pose can help alleviate tension not only in your back but also in your legs and shoulders.

Yoga can be especially beneficial for postpartum mothers who spend a lot of time breastfeeding. These poses can help release tension in the back and hips, improving flexibility and relieving discomfort. One effective pose for this is **Sphinx Pose** (*Salamba Bhujangasana*), a gentle backbend, combined with **Reclining Bound Angle Pose** (*Supta Baddha Konasana*), a hip opener.

Sphinx Pose (*Salamba Bhujangasana*)

1. Begin by lying on your stomach with your legs extended straight behind you, hip-width apart and the tops of your feet pressing into the floor.

2. Place your forearms on the ground in front of you, elbows aligned directly under your shoulders and hands flat on the mat.

3. As you inhale, gently lift your chest off the ground, engaging your lower back muscles. Keep your elbows bent and draw them back towards your ribs, allowing your chest to open forward.

4. Your gaze should be forward or slightly downwards, avoiding the strain of looking up. Keep your lower belly pressing gently into the mat, ensuring that the arch comes from your upper back and not from over-extending your lower spine.

5. Hold for several deep breaths, feeling the stretch along your spine and the gentle opening of your chest.

This backbend is a safe and supportive way to counteract the forward hunching that can come from nursing and is effective in gently strengthening the lower back and stretching your chest and abdominal muscles.

Reclining Bound Angle Pose (*Supta Baddha Konasana*)

1. Start by lying on your back with your legs bent and feet flat on the floor, hip-width apart.

2. Bring the soles of your feet together and allow your knees to fall out to the sides, creating a diamond shape with your legs.

3. Let your arms rest by your sides, palms facing up, or place your hands on your belly or over your heart for added relaxation.

4. Take a deep breath and gently press your knees towards the floor – don't force them down. The focus here is on allowing your hips to open naturally, so feel free to support your knees with pillows or blankets for extra comfort if needed.

5. Stay in this position for at least six rounds of breath, relaxing your back and hips and letting gravity help with the opening of your hips and groin.

When you take a few minutes to release that physical tension, you create space for relaxation, making it easier to engage in the nourishing bond of breastfeeding. I found these small moments of stretching essential in my own journey and continue to do them even today, knowing they help restore balance to my body.

Ultimately, finding a breastfeeding rhythm is about flexibility and self-compassion. You are both learning and growing together and no timetable can dictate the bond you're forming. Embrace the ebb and flow of it all, knowing that each adjustment – whether it's a new sleep pattern, a sudden growth spurt or a change in feeding style – is a part of your journey. Trust yourself, trust your baby and remember that each small step is one of strength, connection and resilience. And as you do this, draw on the practices that help you find peace and balance within yourself, whether through mindful breathing, stretching or simply taking a moment to rest your eyes.

This is not a race, mama. There is no finish line. Embrace the process, as messy and beautiful as it is.

CHAPTER THREE

Managing Your Milk Supply for Nursing and Pumping

The basic principle of breastfeeding is supply and demand. If you breastfeed more often, your body produces more milk to meet your baby's changing needs. If you nurse or pump less, your body will adjust by producing less – sounds so simple, right? When your baby's feeding patterns change, your milk supply will adapt in turn. With this in mind, in this chapter we are going to understand *true low supply* versus *perceived low supply*. So many of the mothers I work with experience anxiety or confusion as their supply naturally fluctuates. I will demystify it for you so that you can understand how you can optimise your supply for your baby. This chapter will also look at pumping, for you pumping mamas who need a more deliberate focus on creating and maintaining your supply without bringing your baby to the boob regularly.

Understanding Milk Supply Changes Over Time

Your milk supply will naturally fluctuate and change at different stages of your breastfeeding journey. During the first few days and weeks, your body is still adjusting, establishing your supply and responding to your baby's demands. But as time passes, many factors come into play that can affect how much milk you produce. This chapter aims to answer some of the common questions I hear from mothers as they move beyond the early stages of breastfeeding. They include:

- How will I maintain my milk supply once I am back at work?

- Do I need to pump overnight if my baby starts sleeping through the night?

- Will my supply remain steady if I get pregnant again?

These questions are all incredibly valid and they reflect the normal ebb and flow of your milk supply as your baby grows, your body heals and your life circumstances change. It's natural for you to feel concerned as your supply adapts, but it's important to know that changes in your milk supply don't necessarily mean there's a problem. On the contrary, it is the adaptability of breast milk – that we touched upon in Chapter One – which makes it so mighty.

Your milk supply is highly influenced by hormones, the frequency of nursing or pumping and your baby's growth and development.

Understanding Low Supply and Oversupply

If you suspect that your milk supply is either too low or too high, it's essential to seek support from a qualified lactation professional, such as an International Board Certified Lactation Consultant (IBCLC) or breastfeeding counsellor. Both are trained to assess your breastfeeding situation and offer personalised solutions for latching, positioning or any other issues that may be affecting your milk supply. Consulting with a lactation specialist can help you pinpoint the root of the issue and find the most effective strategies for managing it.

Identifying Low Milk Supply

Low milk supply is a common concern among breastfeeding mothers, but it's important to determine whether you're truly experiencing low supply or if there's another issue at play. Here are some signs to watch out for:

1. **Your baby seems unsatisfied after feeding:** If your baby is frequently fussy, crying at the breast or appears hungry shortly after feeds, they may not be getting enough milk.

2. **Inadequate weight gain:** Babies should typically gain about 150–200 grams (5–7 ounces) per week in the first few months. If your baby isn't gaining weight as expected, it could indicate they're not receiving enough milk.

3. **Fewer wet and dirty nappies:** From day four to week six, your baby should have 3 or more wet nappies and 5 soft stools per day. Fewer than this may suggest they're not taking in enough milk.

4. **Lack of swallowing sounds:** During feeds, you should hear your baby swallowing regularly. If you don't, it might mean they're not getting much milk.

5. **Breasts feel less full:** If your breasts don't feel fuller before feeds or softer after, this *could* be a sign of low supply (although it is not necessarily).

Steps to Take if you Think you Have a Low Supply

1. **Keep a feeding diary:** Track your baby's feeding patterns, nappy output and behaviour to identify any patterns or concerns.

2. **Monitor weight gain:** Regularly check your baby's weight with your healthcare provider to ensure they're growing as expected.

3. **Assess latch and positioning:** Reach out for an in-person assessment to an IBCLC or breastfeeding counsellor who can provide a thorough latch and positioning assessment.

Identifying True Low Supply vs. Perceived Low Supply

When it comes to breastfeeding, it can feel impossible not to worry about your milk supply, especially as your baby's feeding habits evolve. However, low supply is not always the issue. Many mothers experience moments of doubt, wondering if their milk is enough, particularly as their baby grows and their nursing patterns change. However, not every dip in supply or change in feeding habits signals a problem.

Here are some questions to help you assess whether you're dealing with a true supply issue or if it's more about your perception of your supply:

1. Is my baby gaining weight appropriately?

If your baby is growing steadily, hitting developmental milestones and staying hydrated (i.e. producing enough wet and dirty nappies), chances are your milk supply is absolutely fine. Weight gain is a crucial indicator that your baby is getting enough milk and regular check-ups with your healthcare provider can provide you with reassurance of this.

2. **Is my baby content after most feeds?**

A well-fed baby is generally calm and satisfied after a feed (although this is not necessarily the case if they have a cold or they are teething or otherwise unwell). If your baby seems content, is alert and active when awake and doesn't seem overly fussy or hungry soon after a feed, your milk supply is likely sufficient.

3. **Am I offering both breasts at each feed?**

One of the key factors in ensuring that your milk supply remains strong is offering both breasts during most feeding sessions. If your baby empties both sides during their feed, it's a signal to your body to produce more milk.

If your baby is feeding well from both breasts, it's likely that your milk production is in good shape. When babies drain one breast, it triggers your body to produce more milk and then switching to the other breast promotes a steady supply. This back-and-forth action helps to maintain your overall milk supply, particularly as your baby grows and their nutritional needs increase. Offering both breasts ensures that both sides are being emptied regularly, which in turn supports balanced milk production on each side.

Having said that, it's perfectly normal for some babies to only want one breast per feed. Babies often get a full feed from just one breast, particularly as they become more efficient at nursing. If your baby seems satisfied after nursing on one side and does not seem interested in the second breast when it's offered, there's no need to worry. They're still getting all the nourishment they need. However, if you notice that your baby is consistently only nursing from one breast, it can lead to some imbalances in milk production (and *temporarily* lopsided boobs).

If this is the case, you may find that the breast your baby is not feeding from becomes engorged, while the side that your baby feeds from may be producing more milk. This isn't necessarily a problem, but it could indicate that your milk is not being fully stimulated on both sides. Over time, your body will adjust based on how often each breast is emptied. If you're concerned about your supply or experiencing discomfort from uneven milk production, you could try offering the second breast even if your baby seems full. Alternatively, you could pump the other side after feeds to help maintain balance. Just bear in mind that doing this will increase the amount of milk produced by that breast over time.

Potential Reasons for One-sided Feeding

It's important to consider that your baby may prefer one side due to discomfort or other reasons. Some babies find one breast more difficult to latch onto, or may experience pain which could be related to the birth process. For example, one mother shared that her baby was particularly fretful on one side, and after seeking help from a cranial osteopath, they discovered that the baby was in quite a bit of pain from the birth experience. If your baby consistently refuses one breast or seems uncomfortable, it could be worth exploring different feeding positions to help empty the breast properly with each feed. You might also consider consulting a healthcare professional to ensure there are no underlying issues contributing to your baby's feeding preferences.

If your baby is consistently only nursing on one side, this could signal that your body needs more stimulation to maintain a consistent milk supply. Even if your baby isn't interested in the second breast, simply offering it can help maintain milk production and avoid issues like engorgement or an overactive let-down on the other side.

Also, if your baby is not emptying one side completely, it may lead to milk accumulation in the breast which can cause discomfort and even clogged ducts or mastitis. Offering both breasts consistently can help reduce the risk of these issues and ensure that you maintain a steady supply of milk on both sides. Some people use different tactics to remember which boob they offered last – by clipping a badge onto the side you have just fed after your baby has finished, or swapping a ring or bracelet from one side to the other. You can also simply feel your breasts to distinguish which side you last nursed from, although this may take a little time and practice! These strategies can help with baby brain, making it easier to remember without having to keep track of too many details.

While it's important to offer both breasts, it's equally important to listen to your baby's cues. They know when they're full and will often turn away or stop nursing when they're done. If your baby seems content after nursing on one side and doesn't want more, there's no need to force them to feed from the second breast. On the other hand, if your baby is still rooting around after finishing one side, offering the second breast can help them satisfy their hunger.

As we will discuss in this chapter, it's all about finding the rhythm that works for *you* and *your* baby. Each feeding session is an opportunity to nurture both your baby and your milk supply. The key message here is that your body is adaptable. Over time, your milk production will adjust to your baby's needs, so it's important to stay flexible and trust the process.

I understand how difficult that can be, especially if you are in the throes of postpartum anxiety or depression. I've been there and it is scary. However, you, mama, are the result of millennia of evolution. You stand on the shoulders of generations past – a bridge between history and your baby's future. You are, in every sense of the word, a wonder. Explore the journal exercises on page 106 if you are struggling to tune into your instincts.

4. **Am I experiencing any signs of overproduction (engorgement or forceful let-down)?**

Oversupply can sometimes lead to similar concerns as low supply. If you're dealing with engorgement, frequent leaking or a strong let-down, it could indicate that your supply is more than your baby is currently needing. In such cases, understanding how to manage oversupply might be more important than worrying about low supply. I offer guidance on identifying and managing an oversupply of milk later in this chapter (see page 96).

5. **Is my baby nursing frequently, especially during growth spurts?**

Growth spurts are a completely normal part of your baby's development and they often occur in the first few months. During a growth spurt, your baby may seem suddenly hungrier and demand to nurse more frequently. This increased need for milk is completely natural, as their body is growing rapidly, and they require more nutrition to fuel that growth. While it might feel like your baby is nursing constantly, this is often temporary and should settle down as the growth spurt passes.

6. **Am I feeling stressed or overwhelmed?**

Stress, fatigue and anxiety about breastfeeding can all impact how you *perceive* your milk supply as well as truly affecting your supply. Sometimes, when we're tired or feeling pressure to meet societal expectations, it can feel like you aren't producing enough milk – even when you are. So, if you're experiencing mental or emotional strain, seek support from your family doctor or a mental health professional to address it.

7. **Trust your instincts**

If you have worked through the checklist and everything checks out, but you still have concerns, trust your gut and seek in-person support as soon as possible. If breastfeeding – whether partially or exclusively – matters to you, then it matters that you are empowered to do so.

I hope this checklist leaves you feeling reassured – remember that your body knows what it's doing, so trust the process and be gentle with yourself. If your baby is thriving, your milk supply is more than likely enough. If you're unsure or feel that your supply is truly low, again, please consult in-person with a lactation consultant or healthcare provider to rule out any underlying issues and receive personalised, professional guidance.

Managing Low Milk Supply

If you are experiencing true low milk supply, there are several approaches that, used in combination, can help you maximise the milk you're able to produce. Please remember, each mother's body is unique – what works well for one person might not be the best fit for another. Above all, you deserve to feel supported and empowered in your choices, whatever they may be.

1. Optimise Latch and Positioning

Why it helps: A deep, comfortable latch helps your baby remove milk more efficiently, which in turn signals your breasts to produce more. If the latch is shallow, the breast isn't fully emptied, and your body may not receive the proper cues to keep up milk production.

How to do it: An IBCLC, breastfeeding counsellor or breastfeeding peer supporter can observe you feeding your baby in person or via video consult, suggesting small tweaks to positioning that can make a big difference in milk transfer and comfort. You can also read tips on how to get a good latch in Chapter One of this book (see page 29).

2. Use a Well-fitting, Hospital-grade Breast Pump

Why it helps: If your baby is not able to remove enough milk (due to latch challenges, low or reduced muscle tone or other reasons), or if you're apart from your baby for any reason, pumping can maintain or boost your supply. Hospital-grade pumps are designed for frequent or long-term use and often have better suction patterns to mimic your baby's feeding.

How to do it: Use a nipple-sizer or work with a lactation consultant to ensure that your breast shield/flange size is correct (an incorrect fit can cause discomfort and impede your milk flow). Follow a pumping schedule that stimulates your breasts regularly – ideally matching or slightly exceeding your baby's feeding times.

3. Skin-to-skin Contact and Nursing on Demand

Why it helps: Skin-to-skin contact triggers the release of oxytocin, a hormone that supports let-down and overall milk production. I'm talking full-on, beautiful, naked skin-on-skin. Nursing whenever your baby shows hunger cues ensures that you're optimising that supply-and-demand loop.

How to do it: Try to fit in daily skin-to-skin sessions – even if it's just for a few extra minutes at the end of each feed. Lift your top and your baby's as you breathe them in and snuggle them closely. Offer your breasts often, especially during times your baby is showing early feeding cues (mouth movements, rooting, stirring). Frequent, responsive feeding helps you to maintain the best possible supply.

4. Triple Feeding (Nurse, Pump, Feed Expressed Milk or Supplement)

Why it helps: Triple feeding can temporarily increase stimulation to the breast, helping to boost supply if you suspect that your baby isn't fully emptying your breasts.

How to do it: In a typical session, you'd feed your baby at the breast, then pump immediately after (for 15–25 minutes or as long as is comfortable) and finally offer any expressed milk (or donor milk/formula) to your baby.

Important note: While it can be very effective, triple feeding is an incredibly labour-intensive process. It's not meant to be a permanent routine because the toll on a mother's mental health can be significant. Utilise it short-term and consult with a lactation specialist to determine when and how to scale it back.

5. **Medical Interventions (Domperidone, etc.)**

Why it helps: Domperidone is a prescription medication used in some cases to increase milk supply by raising prolactin levels.
How to use it: If you suspect a hormonal component to your low supply, speak to your GP or a lactation consultant. Domperidone is not suitable for everyone and must be carefully prescribed and monitored. Always discuss potential side effects and any pre-existing conditions with your healthcare provider.

6. **Combination Feeding with Donor Milk and/or Formula**

Why it helps: For some mothers, providing 100 per cent breast milk is not realistic, and combination feeding is a beautifully valid and nurturing option. And yes, you are still breastfeeding if you also choose to offer donor milk or formula.
How to do it: This might involve breastfeeding or pumping at set times, supplemented by donor milk or formula as needed. Some mothers use a supplemental nursing system (SNS) that allows the baby to receive extra milk at the breast, which also stimulates their mother's supply.
Important note: Combination feeding can be a beautifully empowered choice that ensures your baby is well-nourished while you and they continue to benefit from breastfeeding's immunological and emotional advantages.

7. Increase Feeding Frequency

Why it helps: Breastfeeding works on a supply-and-demand basis. The more frequently you nurse or pump, the more signals your body receives to produce milk.

How to do it:

- **Nurse on demand:** Offer the breast whenever your baby shows hunger cues.

- **Include night feeds:** Prolactin levels are higher at night, so feeding during these hours can boost supply.

- **Avoid long gaps between feeds:** Until your baby starts regularly eating solids, try not to let more than three hours pass without feeding or expressing. Bear in mind that it is natural, normal and appropriate for your milk supply to decrease as your baby gradually consumes more and more other food and drinks.

8. Use Breast Compression

Why it helps: During feeds, gently compress your breast to help milk flow more readily. This can encourage your baby to continue feeding and extract more milk.
How to do it: Hold your breast gently but firmly with your fingers around the base and gently squeeze as your baby feeds, helping to move milk towards the nipple.

9. Switch Nursing

Why it helps: Alternate breasts multiple times during a feeding session. When your baby slows down on one side, switch to the other to stimulate more milk production.
How to do it: Offer the second breast after your baby seems to be finished with the first one and switch back and forth until your baby is satisfied and your breasts feel adequately emptied.

10. Avoid Dummies and Bottles (Initially)

Why it helps: In the early weeks, try to meet all your baby's sucking needs at the breast to stimulate your milk supply. Introducing bottles or pacifiers too soon may reduce the amount of time your baby spends breastfeeding.

How to do it: Ideally, it's recommended to wait at least six weeks before introducing a bottle or pacifier. By this time, your baby's latch is likely to be well-established, making it easier to transition between the breast and bottle without affecting your milk supply or feeding routine.

Important note: If you plan to combination feed or exclusively pump from the start, introducing bottles sooner may be necessary. The downside to this approach is that your baby might develop a preference for the bottle, as nursing at the breast is more active and time-consuming for newborns. In contrast, they don't have to work as hard to get milk from a bottle.

A Balancing Act: Supporting Your Mental Health

Managing a true low supply can stir up complicated feelings: sadness, guilt or a sense of loss over the breastfeeding experience you envisioned. It's vital to care for your emotional well-being throughout this process. If methods like triple feeding are taking a toll on your mental health, or if you find yourself feeling consistently overwhelmed, it's okay to pause, reassess and perhaps choose a feeding approach that prioritises both your baby's nutrition and your own well-being.

- **Seek Professional Guidance:** A supportive IBCLC, midwife or doctor can tailor a plan to your unique needs, ensuring that you're not carrying this burden alone.

- **Lean on Your Community:** Whether it's a local breastfeeding support group, online forums or close friends and family, sharing your experiences can alleviate feelings of isolation and remind you that you're not walking this path on your own.

- **Practise Self-compassion:** Remember that your worth as a mother isn't measured by millilitres. The love and care you show – breastmilk, formula or a mixture of both – are what truly count in building a strong, lasting bond with your baby.

If you're facing a truly low milk supply, know that you are *not* failing your baby. Rather, you are doing everything in your power to give them the very best start – often under incredibly challenging circumstances. As I said at the start of this chapter, breastfeeding has never just been about nourishment; it's about forming a secure foundation for your relationship, understanding your own emotional landscape and adapting to new roles as your family evolves. For some mothers that means adapting to topping their baby up with donor milk, combination feeding or formula feeding so that they can be the best possible version of themselves for their families.

No matter what combination of strategies you choose, the magic lies in the connection you foster with your child. Remember that every drop of breastmilk counts and every moment spent cuddling and comforting your baby is a precious part of your journey together. If breastfeeding matters to you – whether you end up exclusively breastfeeding, mixing feeds, or shifting fully to formula – that is what makes your decisions important. Wherever you land, *you* are still the most vital ingredient: a loving mother doing her absolute best.

Potential Causes of True Low Supply

Below are a few of the more common reasons why some women experience true low supply, though this list is by no means exhaustive.

1. **Retained Products of Conception (RPOC)**

What it is: After birth, small fragments of the placenta or other pregnancy-related tissue can sometimes remain in your uterus.
How it affects supply: These retained products can interfere with the body's hormonal signals to produce milk, leading to low supply.
What to do: If you suspect RPOC, it's absolutely vital to consult your healthcare provider for an examination or ultrasound. In many cases, removing the retained tissue can improve your milk production.

2. **Hormonal Imbalances**

What it is: Conditions like polycystic ovary syndrome (PCOS), thyroid disorders (hyperthyroidism or hypothyroidism) and postpartum thyroiditis can all affect milk production.
How it affects supply: Hormones such as prolactin, oestrogen and thyroid hormones play pivotal roles in milk production. An imbalance can disrupt these signals and reduce your milk output.
What to do: When speaking with your doctor, consider asking for:

- Blood tests to check hormone levels, including prolactin, thyroid function (TSH, T3 and T4), oestrogen and progesterone.
- Screening for conditions such as PCOS if you have irregular periods, excessive hair growth or unexplained weight fluctuations.

- A postpartum thyroid function test if you experience fatigue, mood changes or sudden changes in milk supply.

- A referral to an endocrinologist if your results indicate a significant hormonal imbalance that requires specialist care.

- Personalised treatment options such as thyroid medication, dietary changes or managing insulin resistance (in cases of PCOS), which may improve lactation outcomes.

Advocating for these tests and discussions with your healthcare provider can give you a clearer understanding of how your hormones impact breastfeeding and what steps you can take to support your supply.

3. **Breast Surgery or Trauma**

What it is: Past surgical procedures (e.g. breast reduction, augmentation or lumpectomy) or physical trauma to the breast can sometimes damage milk ducts or nerves.

How it affects supply: Any interruption of milk ducts or nerve pathways can hamper a mother's ability to produce or release adequate milk.

What to do: Not all surgeries cause low supply – it depends on the type of procedure and the amount of ductal or nerve involvement. If you have a history of breast surgery, a one-on-one consultation with an IBCLC (International Board Certified Lactation Consultant) can help assess your specific situation and create a tailored plan for you.

4. **Insufficient Glandular Tissue (IGT)**

What it is: Some women have less glandular (milk-producing) tissue in their breasts, a condition sometimes referred to as hypoplasia or IGT.

How it affects supply: Less glandular tissue often translates into reduced milk production capacity (although this is not always the case).

What to do: A proper assessment by a knowledgeable lactation professional is vital. With guidance, many mothers with IGT can still breastfeed – sometimes partially and sometimes fully – by employing specific strategies like frequent feeding, pumping or combination feeding.

5. **History of Infertility with a Hormonal Cause**

What it is: If you experienced any difficulties in conceiving, it's possible those same factors could impact milk production.

How it affects supply: The same hormonal imbalances that affect ovulation and conception might also interfere with the delicate hormonal interplay necessary for producing enough milk.

What to do: Early consultation with an endocrinologist (a hormone specialist) can ensure any hormonal issues are identified and managed, ideally before or early in your breastfeeding journey.

6. **Other Medical Conditions**

What it is: Chronic illnesses, untreated postpartum haemorrhage or certain medications can also reduce milk supply.

How it affects supply: Whether it's due to blood loss, chronic fatigue or side effects of medication, your body may have difficulty sustaining optimal milk production.

What to do: Always inform your doctor of your breastfeeding goals, because alternative medications or specialised support may be available.

Managing your Milk Supply Through Growth Spurts

So, how can you tell if your baby is going through a growth spurt? Growth spurts commonly occur during the first few months of life, particularly around days 3–5, 2–3 weeks, 6 weeks, 3 months and 6 months. However, every baby is unique and these timings vary. Here are a few signs to look out for:

1. **Increased Fussiness and Frequent Nursing:** If your baby seems to be fussier than usual and is wanting to nurse every hour or so, it could be a sign of a growth spurt. Babies may seek the comfort of the breast more often during these periods, not just for nutrition but for comfort as well. They may also seem restless or unable to settle in between feeds.

2. **Shorter, More Frequent Feeding Sessions:** While your baby might be nursing for longer stretches at a time during a growth spurt, you may notice that they want to nurse more frequently, but for shorter periods. This is the body's way of signalling that they need more milk, and as your body works to keep up with the increase in demand, their nursing behaviour adjusts too.

3. **Increased Sleepiness:** Some babies sleep more during a growth spurt to help their little bodies rest and grow. You may notice that your baby is sleeping longer or more frequently overall (woo hoo!), which is completely normal during this time. Once they wake, they will likely want to nurse more.

4. **Changes in Your Baby's Weight and Growth:** Growth spurts are typically followed by noticeable increases in your baby's weight or length. At check-ups, you may notice that your baby has gained weight more quickly than usual. This is perfectly natural and expected. If you feel unsure, a visit to the health visitor or paediatrician can reassure you that the growth is within a healthy range.

5. **Fussiness at the Breast:** During a growth spurt, your baby might seem more frustrated or fussy at the breast, even though they're hungry. They may latch on and off frequently as they try to stimulate more milk production. This can be a sign that they are trying to tell your body that it needs to produce more milk to meet the increased demand.

6. **Changes in Sleep Patterns:** Growth spurts can temporarily disrupt your baby's sleep patterns. They may wake up more frequently at night to nurse or want to cluster-feed in the evenings. This is a normal part of the process and will typically pass once the growth spurt is over.

How to Manage a Growth Spurt

If you're concerned that a growth spurt might be affecting your milk supply, rest assured that this is all part of the beautiful dance between your body and your baby. Your milk supply is perfectly designed to adjust to your baby's ever-changing needs. During a growth spurt, your baby's more frequent nursing will signal your body to produce more milk, so it's important to trust that your body is adapting to meet those evolving demands.

Here's what you can do to help:

- **Offer the Breast More Often:** Let your baby nurse on demand, even if that means more frequent feeds. This will encourage your body to increase milk production to keep up with your baby's needs. Unless you are being advised by a medical or lactation professional, do not limit your baby's nursing sessions; allow them to nurse on demand, for as long as they want.

- **Stay Hydrated and Nourished:** Make sure you're eating well and staying hydrated. Producing milk requires extra energy, so keeping your own body well-fuelled is essential. Read more about breastfeeding and nutrition in Chapter Six (see page 206).

- **Rest as Much as Possible:** Although it may feel like a time of constant feeding, try to rest as much as you can in between. Growth spurts can be tiring for both you and your baby, so if you can, take advantage of nap times to recharge. If you have older children or are back at work, prioritise resting whenever you do get a break or have support at home.

- **Trust the Process:** Trust that growth spurts are temporary even though they feel never-ending at the time. The constant feeding and fussiness will pass, and soon your baby will settle back into a more predictable rhythm. Remember, this is a phase that is helping your baby grow and your milk supply adjust.

Navigating growth spurts, as with so many aspects of breastfeeding and motherhood in general, is about being brave enough to adapt your routine in-line with your baby's nursing behaviour in the knowledge that you, mama, are all that they need.

Consider integrating restful habits into your feeding time. If you're comfy on the sofa, for example, instead of scrunching up and scrolling on your phone, try to incorporate some gentle breathing and softening exercises during your feeding sessions. Unclench your jaw, relax your shoulders and soften your forehead. Notice any tension you might be holding, and consciously release it as you feed. By creating these soothing habits, you can make your feeding time a more mindful and restful experience for both you and your baby.

> **In-the-moment Checklist for Tension**
>
> ♦ Unclench your jaw and relax your face.
>
> ♦ Release any tension in your shoulders, letting them drop away from your ears.
>
> ♦ Soften your forehead.
>
> ♦ Take a few deep, slow breaths, allowing your belly to expand as you inhale and soften as you exhale.
>
> ♦ Check in with your body: are your hands clenched? Your back tight? Release any tension you notice.
>
> ♦ Gently close your eyes if it feels comfortable.

What is Oversupply?

Oversupply occurs when your body produces more milk than your baby needs. This can be due to an overactive milk ejection reflex (let-down) or an abundant milk supply in general. Your body responds to the demand to feed by producing more milk, but sometimes it gets ahead of what your baby can consume. The result? Your baby can feel overwhelmed by the flow, causing gagging, choking, spitting up or difficulty finishing a feed.

If you experience breastfeeding challenges initially, like latch issues or a slow start, your body might overcompensate and produce more milk than necessary. Frequent pumping or pumping more than necessary can also signal to your body to produce extra milk, making it harder to regulate the supply. Other causes include things like excessive stimulation of your breasts, or even external influences, such as stress or hormonal changes. All these factors can trigger your body to overproduce milk, creating a need for your baby to drink more often or in shorter bursts.

You too can feel utterly depleted, as your breasts draw upon your body's reserves of fat, energy and nutrients to maintain your supply. For some mothers, oversupply doesn't always show itself in the immediate early weeks but can develop later. It can be especially difficult to manage when the fast flow of milk causes discomfort or distress to both you and your baby.

Identifying Oversupply

Oversupply might sound like a positive thing, but it can present its own challenges for both you and your baby.

Signs of Oversupply:

1. **Constant engorgement:** Breasts feel overly full or hard – like bowling balls – between feeds. Your baby may seem restless or unhappy at the breast as they struggle to latch onto the firm, round shape of your breasts.

2. **Excessive leaking:** Frequent leaking between feeds, soaking through breast pads.

3. **A forceful let-down reflex:** Your milk sprays or flows rapidly, causing your baby to be overwhelmed by the fast milk flow. They may struggle to keep up with the volume, causing gagging, coughing, or pulling away.

4. **Your baby's behaviour:** Your baby may be gassy, spit up frequently or have green, frothy poos if you have an oversupply of milk.

5. **Frequent spitting up:** If your baby is drinking too much milk too quickly, they may not be able to hold it down, leading to frequent spitting up after feeds.

6. **Frequent blocked ducts or mastitis:** Regular episodes can also indicate oversupply issues.

Steps to Take if you Think you Have an Oversupply of Milk

1. **Observe your feeding sessions:** Note if your baby struggles at the beginning of feeds or seems overwhelmed by the flow of milk.

2. **Monitor your baby's weight gain:** Rapid weight gain can sometimes be a sign of oversupply.

3. **Consult a professional:** An IBCLC or breastfeeding counsellor can assess your situation and confirm if oversupply is the issue.

Managing Oversupply

If you have an oversupply, here are strategies to help regulate your milk production.

1. **Block Feeding**

- **Feed from one breast per session:** Offer only one breast during a feeding to ensure it gets drained well.

- **Extend time on one side:** If needed, feed from the same breast for a set period (e.g. 2–3 hours) before switching to the other side.

This approach helps reduce milk production by allowing the unused breast to become fuller, signalling to your body to slow down the milk-making. By allowing the first breast to empty fully, block feeding reduces the supply on the opposite side. The key hormone involved in this process is dopamine, which is released when the breasts remain full and are not emptied. Dopamine inhibits the release of prolactin, the hormone responsible for stimulating milk production, slowing down your milk production over time.

2. **Adjust Feeding Positions**

- **Laid-back position:** Recline slightly so your baby is nursing 'uphill', which can help slow the flow of milk (see box below for more details on how to get comfy in this feeding position).

- **Side-lying position:** Feeding while lying on your side can also reduce the speed of milk flow (see box below for advice on how to get comfortable in this position).

Laid-back Position

In this position, you lie back comfortably, allowing gravity to help slow the milk flow and giving your baby the ability to latch and feed more easily. Here's what to do:

1. Find a comfortable chair or bed and recline with your upper body supported by pillows. Your body should be at a slight incline, relaxed but supported.

2. Place your baby on your chest, allowing them to rest on their tummy with their head near your breast.

3. Let your baby find the breast themselves, allowing them to latch naturally without any assistance from you. Gravity will help slow down the milk flow, and your baby can nurse at their own pace.

This position is particularly helpful for managing fast let-down and ensuring that your baby is comfortable while feeding.

Side-lying Position

In this position, you and your baby lie on your sides, which can help slow down the milk flow and make feeding more comfortable, especially during times of fast let-down. Here's how to do it:

1. Lie on your side in bed with pillows behind your back for support, ensuring you're comfortable and relaxed. Ensure that there are no pillows or loose sheets anywhere near your baby – and lie on a firm, flat surface such as a bed, mattress or the floor.

2. Position your baby on their side facing you, with their head at the level of your breast. Your baby's body should be aligned with yours, their head slightly tilted and their mouth should be near the nipple.

3. Gently bring your baby close, allowing them to latch onto the breast. You can use your hand to support your baby's back or bottom, but try to avoid holding their head – this can restrict them from latching on naturally.

This position can be especially helpful if you're tired or need a break from sitting up, as it allows for hands-free breastfeeding and makes it easier to nurse in a more relaxed manner. It's also great for managing a fast milk flow, as the horizontal position helps slow the let-down and lets your baby nurse at their own pace.

3. **Manage Your Let-down Reflex**
   - **Express before feeding:** Hand express or pump just enough to relieve initial pressure before latching your baby.

Use gravity: Feed in positions where gravity works against the flow, like laid-back nursing.

4. **Avoid Overstimulation**

- **Limit pumping:** Only pump if necessary for comfort, as pumping can signal your body to produce more milk. If you feel the need to pump, try to avoid pumping immediately after nursing and only if you are feeling uncomfortably full or if you need to build a stash of milk. Try not to wear milk-catchers too often as well.

5. **Gentle Breast Massage:**

- Instead of pumping, you can use gentle breast massage to relieve fullness without stimulating additional milk production. Massage helps to move any stagnant milk towards the nipple and encourages the natural flow of milk, without triggering your body to produce more. This can be particularly helpful if you're feeling engorged or uncomfortable but don't want to increase milk supply.

How to Breast Massage

1. **Position your hands:** Start by placing your hands on your breast, one above your areola (the dark part of your nipple) and one below.
2. **Gentle pressure:** Apply gentle, even pressure as you move your hands in small, circular motions towards the nipple. Start from the outer edges of the breast and work your way towards the centre. This helps to release any milk that might be trapped.

3. **Use your fingertips:** Using the pads of your fingers, gently massage in a rhythmic, circular motion. Start at the outer edges of the breast and work your way towards the nipple, moving in a clockwise or counterclockwise direction. This helps to loosen any tightness in the breast tissue and encourages milk to move towards the nipple without expressing it. You can also try gently moving your fingers in a sweeping motion from the outside of the breast towards the centre. Be sure to apply gentle pressure – there's no need for excessive force, as the goal is to relieve fullness, not to stimulate milk production.

4. **Lift and compress:** You can also try gently lifting and compressing the breast with your hands, moving towards the nipple to help relieve fullness. This helps your milk to flow without the suction that pumping provides.

5. **Avoid overstimulation:** The key is to keep the massage gentle and soothing. Overstimulation can trigger your body to increase milk production, so focus on relieving discomfort rather than trying to express milk.

Massage can be a soothing and effective way to manage fullness without impacting your milk supply. It allows you to relieve pressure and discomfort while keeping your milk production steady.

6. **Controlling the flow**

- **Burp Your Baby Frequently:** Since babies may swallow more air when the milk flows quickly, pause to burp your little one during and after feeds to reduce their discomfort.

- **Pacing the feed:** Allow your baby to nurse in a paced manner, giving them time to swallow and catch their breath. Pausing during the feed to let your baby rest can help them manage the fast flow better and prevent choking or gagging.

7. **Stay Comfortable**

- **Cold compresses:** Apply cold packs or chilled cabbage leaves to your breasts to reduce swelling and discomfort.

- **Wear supportive bras:** A well-fitting, supportive bra can help manage discomfort, but avoid those that are too tight.

- **Diet and hydration:** Sometimes, a balanced diet and staying well-hydrated can help your milk supply stay regulated. But if you have a significant oversupply, over-hydration can contribute to increased milk production.

8. **Monitor for Blocked Ducts and Mastitis**

- Stay vigilant for signs of blocked ducts or mastitis, such as redness, soreness or lumps. If you notice these symptoms, seek medical advice promptly.

One of my clients, Emily, had a significant oversupply. Her breasts were almost permanently engorged, leading to frequent clogged ducts and constant leaking. Her three-month-old baby often choked on the forceful let-down of milk and got sick after every single feed, making feeding stressful for both of them. Unaware that she was exacerbating the issue, Emily was pumping several times a day to relieve her engorgement. This extra pumping signalled to her body to produce even *more* milk.

Working together, we implemented block feeding and adjusted her feeding positions to more laid-back ones. Emily also gradually reduced her pumping sessions, only expressing enough milk to relieve discomfort without emptying her breasts completely. Over time, her milk supply adjusted to her baby boy's needs and feeding became a more comfortable and enjoyable experience for them both.

Seeking Support

Whether you're dealing with low supply or oversupply, remember that you're not alone and help is available. An IBCLC can provide personalised guidance tailored to your situation. Many consultants offer online consultations, so even if local, in-person support isn't accessible, you can still receive expert advice tailored to your particular individual circumstances.

Breastfeeding is a unique journey for you and your baby. It's filled with moments of joy, challenge and learning. By recognising the signs of low supply or oversupply and implementing appropriate strategies, you can navigate these challenges more smoothly. Prioritise self-care, seek support when needed and trust in your body's ability to provide for your baby. With patience and the right guidance, you'll find a rhythm that works for both you and your little one.

For Pumping Mothers

As a pumping mother, you may find yourself navigating a delicate balance – juggling breastfeeding, pumping and the endless responsibilities of caring for a new baby. It can feel like a constant cycle of feeding and expressing milk. In these moments, I want to remind you that pumping remains worthwhile for as long as it feels so for you. Just like breastfeeding, pumping is part of the ebb and flow of your day, especially during those intense cluster-feeding sessions.

Embracing the Rhythm of Pumping and Cluster Feeding

Cluster Feeding

Cluster feeding is when your baby nurses frequently and sometimes seems to 'snack' rather than have full feeds. This can be incredibly physically demanding, however, these moments are key opportunities to maintain your milk supply. If you are nursing alongside pumping, while your baby nurses from your breast, you may need to pump in between sessions to help relieve engorgement or stimulate your milk production. For more detailed guidance on managing your milk supply and pumping techniques, please see page 82. This additional work provides the flexibility to ensure your baby always has access to milk – even when you're not physically present. It allows you to continue nurturing your baby even when you're apart, which is a profound act of love.

That said, the emotional exhaustion that comes with pumping is undeniable. It can sometimes feel like you're living in a cycle of expressing milk, cleaning pump parts and monitoring your output. The mental and physical strain this can cause is nothing short of draining. It's completely normal to feel tired, overwhelmed and at times, even discouraged. Remember, it's okay to acknowledge this fatigue – it's a sign that you're doing the best you can in a demanding situation.

One of the most important things you can do as a pumping mother is to give yourself breaks. While it might feel like every moment is spent either breastfeeding, pumping or cleaning, it's crucial to carve out time for yourself. Acknowledge that you deserve moments to rest and recharge, too. If you can, plan for specific 'pumping breaks' in your day where you can relax. Whether it's curling up with a good book, listening to a podcast or simply enjoying a cup of tea, rather than running errands or getting on with housework as you pump. Doing something small that brings you joy during these breaks can help replenish your energy reserves and make the pumping process feel more manageable.

Navigating the Emotional and Physical Demands of Pumping

Let's talk more about pumping. It's a huge part of the breastfeeding journey for many mothers, whether you're exclusively pumping, combining pumping with breastfeeding or using it as a way to give yourself a break when you need it. But let's be real: pumping is hardly akin to a spa day. On the outside, it might look like an empowering and practical solution to meeting your baby's needs, but behind the pump, it can feel like you're giving even more of yourself then others can see – because you are. Between the physical exhaustion, emotional strain and the constant tracking of milk output, not to mention the constant cleaning and sanitising of pumping parts, it is difficult not to feel overwhelmed. Pumping is far from the flexible solution that many people make it out to be.

Pumping can take a real toll – emotionally and physically. The process itself requires what can feel like bottomless amounts of energy, time and consistency – at a point when your body and mind need more rest than ever. If you're exclusively pumping, the emotional weight of having to be the primary source of nutrition for your baby can feel like a never-ending job. Add to that the physical exhaustion of pumping several times a day and the mental strain of tracking how many millilitres you've managed to express, and it can start to feel like a full-time role on top of every other aspect of mothering. You might find yourself constantly comparing your output to others, wondering if you're producing enough and if you're doing it all 'right'. If this sounds familiar, please, let's take a breath together and acknowledge that you are doing your absolute best, giving your baby your all, and that is more than enough.

It's easy for me to type, 'Don't let the pressure of perfectionism steal your peace!' or 'Cut yourself some slack!', but I know, mama, it's not always that simple. Behind the words of your well-meaning supporters there may be an unrelenting inner critic whispering guilt about not being able to nurse your baby all of the time – or at all. I have lost count of the number of mothers I've worked with who have poured everything they have into providing for their babies, only to beat themselves up for not nursing exclusively, or at all.

I'll never forget an incredibly emotional consultation with Phoebe. Her baby boy, Odin, was 13 months old when she reached out to me for help on how to bring their nursing and pumping journey to a close. But within just a few minutes of our conversation, I could see that Phoebe wasn't anywhere near ready to stop breastfeeding. The issue wasn't that she wanted to stop, but that she couldn't shake the grief of not being able to nurse Odin exclusively, as she had hoped. Like so many mothers I've worked with, Phoebe's journey to parenthood had been shaped by baby loss and infertility. It's a common experience – one that often drives mothers to set impossibly high standards for themselves when it comes to caring for the children they fought so hard for.

During our hour-long chat, I shared with Phoebe how it took me years to come to terms with my own experience of needing an emergency Caesarean section after developing sepsis during labour. It wasn't until my son was three or four years old that I could truly recognise my own dedication and maternal strength. I realised that I had been ready in a heartbeat to put my life on the line in order to bring our baby into the world safely. Similarly, I reminded Phoebe that she had spent countless hours expressing milk for Odin – navigating clogged ducts, battling low supply issues and keeping a constant stream of pump parts washed and sterilised for over a year. Her dedication was beyond measure. It was high time she recognised just how much of herself she was giving to her child.

To put things into perspective, an exclusively pumping mother spends between 120 and 300 minutes per day pumping, especially in the early days. Over the course of a year, that's comparable to a full-time (40-hour-a-week) job! No mean feat. It's an incredibly powerful labour of love, one that deserves just as much recognition as nursing. So, if you are pumping for your baby, partially or exclusively, you are amazing in every sense of the word. That is not to say that any grief you may feel surrounding your breastfeeding journey should be dismissed. It is as real as the love that you feel for your baby and no less valid.

Journal Prompts

Here are some journal prompts to help you recognise your worth as a pumping mama:

1. **Today, I did something incredible for my baby: I pumped.**
   Reflect on how this act, though challenging, is a form of love and dedication. Just one drop of breast milk contains around one million white blood cells. These white blood cells, known as macrophages, help protect your baby from infections.

2. **What is something I've learned about myself through pumping that I never knew before?**
   Maybe it's a new understanding of your resilience, your ability to ask for help or your patience. Take a moment to acknowledge the inner strength you've shown.

3. **When I look at my pumping journey, I see . . .**
   Whether it's a journey of struggle, growth or triumph, reflect on how this experience has shaped you as a mother.

4. **I wish I could tell myself, 'You're doing enough,' because . . .**
   It's so easy to doubt yourself, but remember that you are doing everything you can for your baby. Reflect on what has helped you feel supported and proud, despite the difficulties.

5. **I felt guilty about my pumping today when . . .**
   Write down the moment guilt crept in, and then challenge yourself: what would you say to a friend feeling the same way? You would undoubtedly offer heartfelt compassion and understanding. Do the same for yourself.

6. **Pumping is hard, but it feels worthwhile for my child because . . .**
   Reflect on the emotional weight of pumping. How does the love you feel for your baby fuel your determination, even on the hardest days?

7. **Today, I celebrated a small victory in pumping and it felt . . .**
   Whether it was getting through a pump without stress, reaching a milestone or just taking a moment for yourself afterwards, celebrate the small victories as they matter most.

8. **If my baby could thank me for my efforts today, they would say . . .**

Think about how your baby benefits from your efforts, even if they can't express it yet. What does your love, care and sacrifice mean for them, even in the smallest ways?

9. **Pumping today was emotionally draining, but I want to remember that...**
It's okay to feel drained. Acknowledge the emotional toll it can take, but also remind yourself of the big picture – how it all contributes to your baby's well-being and your own strength.

10. **When I feel exhausted from pumping, what I really need is...**
Tune into your emotional and physical needs. Is it rest, compassion, support or a break? Write about what would make your pumping journey feel a little lighter today. This isn't about reaching for the impossible, it is about tuning into your needs as a pumping mama.

11. **There were moments today when I doubted myself, but I want to remind myself that...**
You're doing your best. Reflect on the moments when self-doubt crept in, but then counter that with something you know to be true about your efforts.

12. **In this moment, I'm going to choose grace. I'll remind myself that...**
Give yourself permission to let go of perfection. It's okay if things aren't perfect or if the output isn't what you wanted today. What matters is the incredible effort you've made, and the love behind it.

The Rewards of Pumping

Having acknowledged some of the challenges, it's also true that pumping can be deeply rewarding. There's something incredibly empowering about knowing you're providing nutrition for your baby – irrespective of whether they're nursing directly from your breast. Each millilitre of milk you pump is a victory. It's a tangible reminder of your body's incredible ability to nourish your little one, even if the process doesn't always feel easy or natural. And of course, pumping does offer some flexibility. It can give you the space to take a break or let someone else help with feeding while you rest, recover or just have a moment for yourself. It might not always feel effortless, but it is an important part of your motherhood journey, and it's something to be incredibly proud of.

For many mothers, pumping can offer a strong sense of purpose. It might feel like a challenging task, but with it comes the knowledge that you're doing everything you can for your baby's well-being. There's a quiet bonding moment when you pump, knowing that every drop of milk is a gift for your baby. Even though pumping might not involve the same physical connection as direct breastfeeding, it still serves the same purpose of nourishment, love and connection. Your effort is building a foundation for your baby's growth, and that in itself is deeply meaningful.

Practical Tips for Managing Pumping

Let's start by setting small, achievable goals. It's easy to get caught up in the idea of pumping the 'perfect' amount, but instead, focus on what works for you and your baby. Aim for consistency, not perfection. For instance, try to pump at the same time each day so it becomes part of your routine and give yourself permission to miss a session or adjust if needed. It's okay if the milk output doesn't look the same every time – each session is still important, and so are you! There will undoubtedly be days when your baby sleeps a longer stretch than usual, and you skip a pumping session in favour of a few more moments of shut-eye. Don't beat yourself up for being human; give yourself some recognition for choosing self-love when you need it.

A seldom-discussed but crucial tip for pumping is to label any expressed milk as being pumped during the day or overnight. This is important because overnight, your milk contains sleep-inducing hormones (melatonin and cholecystokinin, or CCK) to help your baby establish their circadian rhythm. Milk expressed in the morning, on the other hand, contains more of the stress hormone cortisol, which helps your baby feel more alert and awake during the day – not exactly what you want at 2am!

In the early days, don't be afraid to ask for help. If you're feeling drained (no pun intended), see if someone can take over baby care for a short while so you can focus on pumping without the extra distractions. And be kind to yourself – pumping is a skill, just like breastfeeding. It takes practice, patience and time to get into a rhythm. Here are some tips to help you get your pumping journey off to the best possible start.

Choosing a Pump

For some mothers, the thought of pumping can feel daunting, but it's important to remember that finding the right pumping tool can make the process a little easier and more comfortable. There are several options available, each with its own set of benefits and drawbacks. Whether you are looking to pump frequently, collect milk in between feeds or express on the go, there is something to suit your needs. Let's look at a few options that might work for you.

Milk Catchers

Often used in combination with breastfeeding, milk catchers are a great tool to help collect milk that would otherwise be lost during a feed. These small, lightweight devices fit comfortably in your bra and catch any milk that leaks from the opposite breast while you nurse or pump. They are especially helpful if you experience let-down – when your milk starts to flow – from the non-nursing breast and want to capture the milk without having to manually pump or waste it. Milk catchers are a fantastic choice for building a stash without the effort of additional pumping sessions.

Benefits:

- Gentle on your body and simple to use.
- Can be worn during feeding, allowing you to collect milk without interruption.
- Discreet and portable, great for mothers who want to save milk without extra effort.
- Ideal for light to moderate milk leakage.

Drawbacks:

- May not be ideal if you're looking to collect larger quantities of milk.
- Not a good option for exclusive pumping, as they are not designed for stimulating milk production over longer periods.
- Could inadvertently cause an oversupply of milk (remember that the more milk is removed from your breasts the more milk your breasts will produce).

Silicone Suction Breast Pumps

Silicone suction pumps are manual, non-electric pumps that create gentle suction to draw out milk from the breast. These pumps are often praised for their simplicity, portability and quiet operation. They are easy to use and can be used alongside nursing or separately.

Benefits:

- Gentle and effective for occasional pumping, especially if you're looking to express a little extra milk during or after feeds.

- Silent, discreet and easy to clean, making them ideal for on-the-go pumping.

- No need for batteries or electricity.

- Lightweight and portable – ideal for pumping in between nursing sessions without needing to set up anything complicated.

Drawbacks:

- Can take longer to express milk compared to electric pumps.

- Not the best option if you need to pump regularly or in large amounts.

Manual Breast Pumps

Manual breast pumps are another popular choice and require you to pump by hand. These pumps usually consist of a handheld unit with a handle you squeeze to create suction. While they can be slightly more labour-intensive, they offer full control over the suction and can be incredibly effective when used correctly. They are a solid option for mothers who want something affordable and more robust than a milk catcher but without the complexity of an electric pump.

Benefits:

- Provides full control over suction strength and speed, allowing you to find a rhythm that works for you.

- Compact and portable, with no need for electricity or batteries.

- Easy to clean, as there are often fewer parts compared to electric pumps.

- Great for occasional use, or for mothers who want a reliable, manual option when electric pumps aren't available.

Drawbacks:

- Can be physically tiring, especially if you are pumping frequently.

- Time-consuming – manual pumping generally takes longer than using an electric or wearable pump.

- May not be suitable for exclusive pumping or when needing to pump multiple times a day.

Electric Breast Pumps

Electric pumps are often the go-to choice for mothers who need to pump regularly or want to express large quantities of milk efficiently. They are fast, effective and usually come with a range of settings to mimic a baby's nursing pattern. These pumps often offer the flexibility of double-pumping, too.

Benefits:

- Fast and efficient – ideal for mothers who need to pump frequently or build a milk supply quickly.
- Double pumping options help save time by expressing milk from both breasts at once.
- Adjustable settings to help you customise suction and speed for comfort.
- Many models come with timers, app controls and memory settings that make the process easier to track and adjust.

Drawbacks:

- Larger and bulkier than manual or silicone pumps, which might not be ideal for travelling.
- Can be noisy, which may be a concern for you.
- The initial investment can be higher compared to manual or silicone pumps.

Wearable Pumps

Wearable pumps are a more recent innovation, providing the ultimate in flexibility. They are small, discreet and worn inside your bra, allowing you to pump hands-free while going about your day. Though they are not as powerful as traditional electric pumps, they provide an incredible amount of freedom for mothers who need to express on the go or while multitasking.

Benefits:

- Hands-free and portable – ideal for expressing milk while doing other tasks, like working, cleaning or spending time with family.
- Silent and discreet, so you can pump without others noticing.
- Lightweight and easy to move around with.
- Convenient for mothers who want to pump while caring for their baby.

Drawbacks:

- Generally less powerful than traditional electric pumps, which may mean pumping takes longer or requires more frequent sessions.
- They might encourage multitasking, which isn't always helpful, especially when you need to focus on resting or caring for yourself.
- Not recommended for mothers who want to exclusively pump, as they may not be powerful enough to build a full milk supply.

Choosing the right pump for you is an incredibly personal decision. You might try a few different types before you find the one that fits your lifestyle and meets your needs. Remember, whether you're using a milk catcher, silicone pump, manual pump or electric pump, there is no one 'right' way to express milk. The most important thing is that you're taking care of yourself while meeting your baby's needs, and that is a huge accomplishment.

Pumping Tips

Before

1. Check your flange/shield size of your pump. Is it comfortable? Your nipple should fit flush against the flange/shield, filling it without any rubbing as you pump. As a guide you should measure the base of your nipple and then add 3–5mm to find your correct flange size. Some manufacturers include various breast shield sizes with the pump, whilst others do not.

2. Take a drink and some snacks with you as you prepare to pump. Although there is no direct link between adequate hydration and milk output (unless you are severely dehydrated); this step is simply about looking after yourself, mama.

3. Gently massage, tap or knead your breasts, starting below your armpits in circular motions moving towards your nipples for a few minutes before you start pumping.

4. Do a few rounds of deep breathing before you start. Doing so will calm your parasympathetic nervous system, getting your body and mind ready to pump.

During

1. Keep your baby close or look at photos or videos of them to get that oxytocin flowing and to help induce a let-down as you pump. Turn up the volume on any videos for maximum effectiveness.

2. Flood your sense receptors with your baby by smelling one of their worn items of clothing.

3. Listening to your favourite songs may help you to get your body and mind ready for that liquid gold to

flow, too. Choose music that you have an emotional connection to for best results.

4. Cover your pump so that you cannot see how much milk you are pumping at any given time. This will help you to be as calm and relaxed as possible, maximising your milk output.

5. If you are using an electric pump, use the expression mode on your pump (if there is one) at the beginning of a pumping session to mimic the shorter, faster sucks that your baby does when they nurse at the start of a feed. You can echo this with a manual pump by doing shorter, quicker pumps at the start of your pumping session. Once your let-down happens, slow your manual pumps down, holding the handle of the pump down for a few seconds at a time. If you are pumping to build your supply by emptying your breasts, pump for 25–30 minutes if possible and comfortable.

After

Change your pump parts frequently as per manufacturer guidelines, so that you know that your pump is working as effectively as possible.

Staying Hydrated

Investing in a water bottle that can be opened with one hand is a simple but valuable tip. If you are pregnant as you read this, it will be useful during labour as well as after birth. Many of us have heard that the human body is approximately 60 per cent water, but did you know that breast milk is around 90 per cent water? Staying well-hydrated can make everything feel just a little more manageable – a benefit you may notice even more when you are sleep-deprived and recovering from childbirth. Dehydration can make you feel depleted and irritable and may even affect your milk production.

For some mothers, dehydration can even trigger nursing aversion. This aversion can manifest as feelings of agitation, frustration or even anger during breastfeeding, as if your body is signalling that it's lacking the hydration required for lactation. The science behind this is tied to your body's stress response. When you're dehydrated, your body goes into a mild state of stress and this can increase cortisol levels – the stress hormone. High cortisol levels can interfere with the release of prolactin, which makes breastfeeding feel more difficult or uncomfortable.

I remember experiencing this during the second year of our breastfeeding journey; I was dumbfounded when I realised that it was my struggle to prioritise my own hydration that was making nursing my then-toddler feel so much more challenging. It wasn't just about feeling thirsty – it was my body reacting to dehydration, making the whole experience feel more tense and less rewarding. This was a real eye-opener for me and it highlighted just how essential it is to care for yourself in the same way you care for your baby, especially when it comes to staying hydrated. When you're properly hydrated, not only does it support your milk supply, but it also helps calm your nervous system and ease the physical and emotional strain that can come with breastfeeding.

There is no need to worry about drinking vast quantities of water each day: the best advice is simply to drink 'to your thirst'. In reality, like many of my clients, you may find it challenging to stay in tune with your body's cues amid the demands of new motherhood. A useful target can be to drink an additional 700ml to 1 litre each day (roughly two or three average-sized tumblers) on top of the usual recommended 2 litres. Individual needs do vary based on factors like height, weight and metabolism, so treat these figures as flexible guidance rather than a strict rule.

One practical tip that helped me manage my water intake was to have a drink each time I nursed my son. I did not follow this religiously once he began eating solid foods and drinking other liquids, but in the early days, it helped me avoid headaches and maintain energy. Keep a large glass or bottle by your bed and drink the whole thing before you get out of bed in the morning. This technique draws upon the ideas of habit stacking – linking something that you *want* to do (drink more water), with something that you *must* do (get out of bed). Making self-care habitual literally removes the need to think about it from the equation, leaving you free to focus on loving your baby.

> *A note of caution: it is possible to overdo hydration, and excessive water intake is neither beneficial for you, nor your milk supply. Listen to your body, stay in tune with your natural thirst cues and approach hydration with balance.*

Eating to Support Yourself and Your Baby During Breastfeeding

Breastfeeding affects your hunger and appetite in complex ways. You require additional calories – 450–500 extra per day, depending on your metabolism and activity levels. Breastfeeding can cause your blood sugar levels to drop, often triggering intense hunger pangs. Hormonal changes play a significant role in regulating your appetite. Ghrelin, commonly known as the 'hunger hormone', tends to be released at higher levels when you're sleep-deprived, and as breastfeeding often involves frequent overnight waking, elevated ghrelin levels can lead to feeling completely ravenous. The hormonal shifts that suppress oestrogen and progesterone during breastfeeding can either amplify or dampen appetite, with the effects varying depending on individual circumstances, stress levels and overall health.

Keep Snacks Nearby

Keeping snacks close by is a game-changer when you get the feeding munchies. We all know that the demands of nursing can trigger intense hunger pangs at the most unexpected times – often in the middle of the night when you're feeling utterly drained. Having a selection of snacks at your fingertips makes all the difference. Ideally, these should be nourishing rather than sugar-laden, although let's be honest, the occasional treat can be a much-needed comfort during those long sessions. Granola bars, dried fruit and chocolate-coated peanuts are great options to keep in the baby change bag or within arm's reach on the coffee table. Yoghurt, fresh fruit, rice cakes, energy balls and cereal bars are also fantastic go-tos that are easy to grab when you're focussed on feeding your little one.

To make sure your snacks are always fresh and ready to go, consider storing them in sealable containers or small, portable tubs that you can take with you throughout the day. If you love hummus, it's a wonderful, protein-packed option that requires no preparation and can be eaten with just one hand while you're nursing. For a nutritious twist, you can blend store-bought hummus with peas, carrots or beetroot for added variety and a burst of flavour.

Protein is a vital nutrient when you're breastfeeding. Not only does it support milk production, but it also aids in your body's recovery after birth. Incorporating protein-rich foods – such as lean meats, eggs, dairy, legumes and nuts – helps meet the increased demands your body faces during this special time. Studies have shown that a sufficient intake of protein enhances the quality of your milk, boosting the production of key immunological proteins essential for your baby's immune system. Additionally, protein-packed snacks throughout the day can help stabilise your blood sugar levels, which can fluctuate while breastfeeding, pumping or expressing milk. By keeping your energy levels steady, these snacks ensure you feel nourished and ready to take on the world – one feed at a time.

Bonus tip: ask your partner or a family member to help keep your snack supply topped up each week. It's a small task that can make a big difference, and it means you won't have to worry about preparing snacks yourself during those precious, quiet moments. By delegating this responsibility, you'll always have something healthy and nourishing close at hand, without the added stress of having to plan and prepare it yourself.

Can Snacks Actually 'Boost' Lactation?

The idea of lactation-boosting snacks is a bit controversial among medical and lactation professionals. While many mums report anecdotally that certain foods and drinks seem to help their milk supply, the only proven, non-medical methods for boosting milk production are ensuring you get enough rest, staying hydrated, eating balanced meals and frequently emptying your breasts. Breastfeeding operates on a supply-and-demand basis – nursing or pumping more often signals to your body to produce more milk, while less frequent milk removal can lead to a decrease in supply.

Managing your pumping journey requires a balance of dedication, self-care and patience. As we've explored, staying hydrated, fuelling your body with nourishing snacks and creating a routine that works for you are all ways to honour the profound work you're doing. Pumping may not always feel effortless, but it is an extraordinary act of love – a quiet, steadfast way of nourishing your baby, even when you're apart.

Every drop of milk you produce is a testament to your strength, resilience and unwavering care for your little one. It's a powerful reminder that, even in the most demanding moments, you are giving a piece of yourself to help your baby thrive. So, as you continue on this journey, remember that you are creating something truly beautiful, woven together with love, sacrifice and tenderness.

Take time to rest, nurture your own needs and embrace the journey with grace – because the love you pour into your baby, through every feed and every moment, is a love that transcends the challenges.

CHAPTER FOUR

Troubleshooting – Thriving Through the Challenges

Breastfeeding has never *just* been about feeding our babies – it's about building the foundations of a lifelong relationship, navigating your emotions (and your baby's) and learning how to balance your new role as a mother with the needs of your growing family. The early days and months are often full of challenges – way more than most of us anticipate – but with patience, self-compassion and a little guidance, these difficulties can become opportunities for truly transformative growth and connection.

As you find your way through the ups and downs of breastfeeding, it's crucial to remember that challenges are a normal part of the process. These obstacles – such as low milk supply, oversupply, nursing strikes, teething and sleep deprivation – can feel completely overwhelming when you are in the midst of them. But with the right support, tools and mindset, you *can* overcome them – they don't have to define your nursing or pumping journey. It is the greatest privilege to be able to guide you through these common hurdles, offering practical solutions and, most importantly, reassurance that you are not alone on this path.

Hormonal Changes

In the early weeks, the hormone prolactin plays a crucial role in establishing your milk supply. Prolactin stimulates milk production, ensuring your body produces enough milk to meet your baby's growing needs. Meanwhile, oxytocin helps your milk flow by triggering the let-down reflex, allowing your baby to access the milk. Over time, as your baby's feeding patterns change – such as when they start sleeping for longer stretches or if you return to work – your body adjusts the amount of milk it produces based on demand. This process is driven by a feedback loop of hormones: the more milk that is removed from your breasts (either by breastfeeding or pumping), the more prolactin is released, signalling to your body to produce more milk.

Conversely, if milk is not removed as frequently, prolactin levels decrease, leading your body to produce less milk. This is the body's natural way of responding to your baby's changing needs. I dedicate a whole chapter of this book to navigating your return to work, and for more help and support with that, head to Chapter Eight (see page 227).

Oral Ties: Understanding and Addressing Tongue and Lip Ties

One of the less visible but incredibly common challenges is the issue of oral ties – often referred to as tongue-tie or lip-tie. Many of my clients around the world had never even heard of oral ties before they found themselves battling severe nipple pain, cracked nipples and mastitis. Undiagnosed lip and tongue-ties cause so many mothers so much unnecessary pain and difficulty. This is why I want to take a moment to talk about oral ties, their impact on breastfeeding, and how they can affect both you and your baby.

What Are Oral Ties?

Oral ties, also known as tethered oral tissues (TOTs), refer to the condition where the tongue or lip's frenulum (the piece of tissue that connects the tongue or lip to the mouth) is either too tight or restrictive. This can cause breastfeeding difficulties, such as a shallow latch, nipple pain or inefficient milk transfer. Tongue-tie occurs when the frenulum under the tongue is too short or thick, restricting the tongue's range of motion. A lip-tie happens when the frenulum connecting the upper lip to the gums is too tight, limiting the lip's ability to flange outwards properly during feeding. Not all babies with oral ties experience breastfeeding issues, but for many mothers, it can be a significant barrier to establishing a comfortable and effective feeding relationship.

How Can Oral Ties Affect Breastfeeding?

Oral ties can cause tension while nursing, regardless of whether your baby is attaching well or not. If your baby has oral ties there is often a noticeable tension during feeding. This tension can cause discomfort for both you and your baby, making breastfeeding feel stressful instead of the bonding experience it could be.

Some of the common signs and symptoms to look out for include:

- **Nipple pain and damage:** Nipple pain that doesn't resolve with good positioning or that persists despite efforts to improve latch may be a sign of an oral tie. Many mothers describe the pain as a sharp or burning sensation, often coupled with cracked or blistered nipples.
- **Shallow latch:** If your baby is struggling to latch deeply or feed effectively, they may not be getting enough milk,

which can lead to insufficient weight gain or excessive hunger between feeds. A shallow latch can often be linked to oral ties. Babies with a shallow latch often struggle to get enough milk, leading to frustration for both mother and baby.

- **Frequent or long feeds:** Babies with tongue or lip ties may feed for long periods without appearing satisfied. They often fall asleep quickly at the breast due to inefficient sucking, which can lead to overfeeding or frustration from the mother when milk isn't being transferred properly.

- **Excessive gas or reflux-like symptoms:** Air intake from a poor latch can lead to gassiness, colic or even reflux. Babies may appear uncomfortable during or after feeds, as they swallow air along with milk.

- **Mastitis and clogged ducts:** When milk isn't being removed effectively due to a poor latch, it can lead to engorgement and blockages in the milk ducts, which can increase the risk of mastitis or clogged ducts.

Addressing Oral Ties: What You Can Do

If you think that your baby may have an oral tie, it's important to seek support from an IBCLC or a healthcare professional experienced in assessing and diagnosing oral ties. A thorough assessment is essential, as oral ties can be complex and vary widely in severity.

Things you can do/go to an expert and get checked:

1. **Latching and positioning:** If your baby is experiencing difficulty latching due to an oral tie, a lactation consultant can help you work on improving the latch. Sometimes,

small adjustments in positioning can make a big difference, even if an oral tie is present.

2. **Suck-training exercises:** These exercises are designed to help your baby learn to use their mouth and tongue more effectively. They can also help strengthen the muscles necessary for proper latching and feeding. It's important that these exercises are done alongside support from an International Board Certified Lactation Consultant (IBCLC), who has assessed your baby in person. The exercises are most effective when they are tailored to your baby's unique and specific needs, so it's crucial to get professional guidance.

3. **Manual oral exam:** This will assess your baby's tongue and lip function and help determine the severity of the tie and whether further intervention is needed.

4. **Seeking treatment for oral ties:** In some cases, an oral tie may need to be released to allow better tongue or lip mobility. This can be done through a simple procedure, often referred to as a frenotomy or frenectomy, which involves snipping the restrictive frenulum. This can be carried out by a paediatrician or an experienced provider who is skilled in infant oral assessments. If this treatment is chosen, working with an IBCLC before and after the procedure is vital to ensure breastfeeding continues smoothly and to protect your milk supply.

5. **Gentle bodywork:** If there's a history of a difficult birth, a baby may have tension or misalignment in their head and neck that affects feeding. Gentle cranial osteopathy or chiropractic care, when performed by a qualified professional, can help release tension in these areas and support better feeding patterns.

Support is Key: Don't Struggle Alone

Dealing with oral ties can be frustrating, especially when you feel like you've tried everything but are still facing challenges. Please know that you are not alone. So many of the mothers I have worked with have faced similar difficulties and have gone on to establish successful, pain-free breastfeeding relationships after addressing the issue. They were successful because they sought help, instead of thinking that they had to figure it out alone.

Self-compassion is vital too: it's easy to feel like you're failing or doing something wrong, especially when you may have received conflicting advice. Give yourself permission to be a beginner and remember that finding the right support is a step towards a positive change. Every breastfeeding journey is unique, and just because things aren't going smoothly right now doesn't mean you won't find a solution that works for you and your baby.

Sometimes, addressing oral ties can be an ongoing process, but for as long as it matters to you, the reward of a comfortable, effective breastfeeding relationship is worth the effort. Rely on your body's ability to nurture your baby, and trust that with the right support, you can work through these challenges together.

Coping with Colic

Nothing is more distressing than seeing your baby in pain and feeling completely helpless. The term 'colic' is often used to describe periods of excessive crying or discomfort in babies, but it's important to note that it is not a medical diagnosis. Rather, colic refers to a pattern of unexplained crying or distress, typically in an otherwise healthy baby, where no other medical issues are identified. This can make it even more frustrating, as there may not be a clear cause and the crying can feel relentless.

Many parents have been through the turmoil of colic, and while it can be one of the most challenging aspects of the early months, it's important to remember that it is a phase that will eventually pass. The good news is that, as your baby's loving caregiver, you are the one who can help soothe them and provide comfort during this time. By offering your nurturing presence and patience, you can make all the difference in easing your baby's discomfort and maintaining your own sense of control, even in the most difficult moments.

Colic is thought to be caused by several factors, including digestive discomfort, sensitivity to milk or even overstimulation. While the exact cause remains unclear, it's important to remember that colic is not your fault and it doesn't mean you're doing anything wrong as a parent. The good news is that colic is temporary. It usually peaks at around 6–8 weeks and tends to improve significantly by 12–16 weeks, with many babies outgrowing it entirely by 4–6 months.

Signs of colic include:

- **Excessive crying:** Colic typically presents as intense crying spells, often in the late afternoon or evening, which can last for more than three hours a day, three or more days a week.

- **Fussiness:** Colicky babies often seem difficult to soothe, even when fed, changed or held. They may pull their knees towards their chest or make fists, showing discomfort.

- **Gassiness:** Some babies with colic may also experience gas or seem to have trouble passing wind, which can contribute to their crying.

- **Unpredictability:** Colic tends to come in waves, with your baby seeming perfectly calm one moment and crying inconsolably the next.

How Does Colic Relate to Breastfeeding?

It's easy to feel as though colic is somehow connected to breastfeeding, especially if your baby seems to cry more after feeding or appears fussy during breastfeeding. However, while colic can occur in both breastfed and formula-fed babies, breastfeeding can sometimes offer some relief. The close contact, soothing motions and comfort of your milk can be reassuring to your baby during these difficult episodes.

That said, there are some breastfeeding-related issues that can contribute to or exacerbate colic-like symptoms. For example:

- **Oversupply:** If you have an oversupply of milk, your baby might be overwhelmed by the forceful let-down, leading to gassiness or difficulty latching properly. This could contribute to discomfort.

- **Milk sensitivity or intolerance:** Some babies may have sensitivities to certain proteins or components in breast milk, often related to dairy products, or other foods in your diet.

- **Swallowing air during nursing:** A poor latch can lead to your baby swallowing air, which can cause gassiness and discomfort.

If you think your baby's colic may be related to something in your diet or their feeding habits, it might be worth seeking the advice of a lactation consultant to assess your milk supply, latch and your baby's feeding pattern. Sometimes even small adjustments can make a real difference to your baby's comfort.

Ways to Alleviate Colic

1. **Check your baby's latch:** If your baby is swallowing a lot of air during feeds, it could be causing discomfort. An IBCLC can help you assess your baby's latch and make sure they are feeding effectively and comfortably.

2. **Manage oversupply and forceful let-down:** If you're dealing with oversupply, block feeding (feeding from one side per session for a few feeds in a row) or other strategies may help manage milk flow (see page 96 for advice on block feeding). Slower, more frequent feeds can reduce the chances of your baby becoming overwhelmed.

3. **Burp often:** Gassiness can exacerbate colic, so make sure to burp your baby during and after feeds. Sometimes the simple act of getting rid of trapped air can make a world of difference.

4. **Create a calm environment:** Colic can be exacerbated by overstimulation. During these episodes, try to reduce noise and bright lights. Some babies find it comforting to be swaddled when not feeding, held close or rocked gently.

5. **Try gentle tummy massage:** Some parents find that gentle tummy massages can help relieve gas and soothe their baby. One technique that many find helpful is the 'I Love You' massage, which you can find described in the box on the next page. This involves gently tracing the letters 'I', 'L' and 'U' on your baby's tummy with your fingers. These movements help to stimulate digestion and release trapped gas.

6. **Consider an elimination diet:** If you suspect that your baby's colic might be related to something in your diet (such as dairy or other allergens), consider eliminating these foods and tracking any changes in your baby's

behaviour. Please always consult a healthcare professional before making dietary changes.

7. **Soothing techniques:** White noise, gentle rocking, swaddling or a warm bath can help calm your baby. What works may vary from one baby to the next, but keeping a variety of soothing options available can help you feel more in control.

To perform the 'I Love You' massage:

- **I:** Start by gently stroking your baby's tummy from the top of their belly, down to the bottom on the left side of their body (following the shape of the letter 'I').

- **L:** Next, trace an 'L' shape on their tummy, starting from the left side and moving across their tummy and down towards the right side.

- **U:** Finally, trace a 'U' shape by gently sweeping from the left side of the tummy, around the bottom, and back up the right side.

There are lots of videos and detailed guides online to help you learn the technique and to ensure that you're doing it gently and effectively.

When to Seek Help

If your baby's crying is accompanied by other concerning symptoms, such as a fever, vomiting or refusal to feed, it's important to seek medical advice. A health professional can rule out other conditions, such as reflux, allergies or infections that may be contributing to your baby's discomfort.

I understand just how tough colic can be. The constant crying, the sleepless nights that seem to stretch on endlessly and the feeling of not knowing how to soothe your baby – it's incredibly hard. Please, know that you are doing an incredible job. You are your baby's world, and every step you take to comfort and calm them matters deeply. The colic phase will eventually pass and in time, you'll look back on this difficult season with the understanding that you faced it with resilience, patience and boundless love.

No, this is not easy and there is no 'right' way to handle it, but remember – you can do hard things, especially with the right support. It's okay to feel overwhelmed; it's okay to ask for help. You are not alone in this. If the crying is taking a toll on you or you find yourself at a breaking point, please don't hesitate to reach out for support. Cry-sis is a charity dedicated to supporting parents of babies with excessive crying – they can offer you guidance and a compassionate ear. Find more information at Cry-sis.org.uk. Asking for help is not a sign of weakness; it's a sign of strength.

Please, give yourself credit for all the love and care you are giving your baby, even on the toughest days. You are doing the best you can and that is all any of us can ever do.

Reflux

I had heard of reflux before my son was born, but I had no real understanding of just how much it would affect our lives in those early months. When my son was a newborn, breastfeeding felt like a chaotic whirlwind at times. He was nursing well, and after a rocky start to our breastfeeding journey, he was gaining weight as expected. However, what I didn't realise at the time was that I had inadvertently created an oversupply of milk, which meant my let-down was like a fire hose. Every time my son nursed he was bombarded with a gush of milk. At first, he didn't seem to mind this fast flow and I was grateful that he was feeding well. But after a few weeks I noticed that after every feed, if he wasn't held upright for at least 30 minutes, he would be sick. This wasn't a huge issue during the day, but when it happened in the middle of the night, with feeds stretching for 45 minutes or more, it became unbearable. My partner and I lived like zombies, desperately trying to get through each sleepless night as a tag team. Caring for our rainbow baby boy was everything we had hoped for, but it also drained us completely. What I didn't realise then was that the combination of fast let-down and oversupply was likely causing his reflux, making everything so much harder.

What is Reflux?

Reflux, also known as gastro-oesophageal reflux, is a common condition in infants where milk flows back up from the stomach into the oesophagus. This happens because the valve between the stomach and the food pipe is not fully mature in newborns, causing milk to return upwards. This can lead to spitting up and, in some cases, discomfort for your baby.

It's important to distinguish between spitting up and vomiting. Spitting up is a normal and common occurrence in infants, typically happening after or during feeding. It usually involves a small amount of milk that your baby brings up and it's typically a gentle regurgitation. Spitting up is not usually a cause for concern, especially if your baby is feeding well, gaining weight and seems content otherwise.

On the other hand, vomiting is different. It often involves a larger amount of milk coming up forcefully and may be accompanied by distress or discomfort. Vomiting can sometimes be a sign of an underlying issue, such as an infection or more severe reflux, so if your baby is vomiting frequently or seems to be in pain, it's important to speak with a healthcare professional to rule out any concerns.

For many babies, reflux and spitting up are completely normal and resolve on their own as they grow and their digestive system matures. Like us, by the time your baby is six months old, you may notice their symptoms begin to lessen. Most babies will have outgrown reflux by their first birthday, as the valve between the stomach and food pipe becomes stronger.

What Causes Reflux?

In the early days, reflux can be caused by several factors and sometimes it's a combination of these. The most common causes of reflux in infants include:

- **Immature sphincter muscles:** The valve that keeps milk in the stomach is still developing, which means it doesn't always do its job properly.

- **Oversupply or fast let-down:** If you have a fast-flowing milk supply or an overactive milk ejection reflex (let-down), your baby may struggle to cope with the rapid flow, causing milk to back up into your baby's oesophagus.

- **Air intake during feeding:** If your baby is not latching deeply or is gulping air while feeding, it can lead to discomfort and reflux.

- **Other factors:** Conditions like oral-ties, allergies or even the position in which your baby is fed can also trigger reflux.

For me, the fast let-down and oversupply were key factors in my son's reflux. But the good news is that reflux is often a phase that improves with time. As your baby's digestive system matures, the frequency and severity of reflux episodes will likely reduce.

How to Manage Reflux in Your Baby

There are several ways to help ease your baby's discomfort during this phase.

- **Upright positioning after feeds:** Try to keep your baby upright for 30 minutes after feeds to help milk stay down. This can be a challenge, especially during night feeds, but it can make a significant difference.

- **Shorter, more frequent feeds:** Instead of longer feeding sessions, try offering shorter, more frequent feeds to prevent your baby from overloading their stomach.

- **Correcting latch issues:** If your baby is struggling with a poor latch, it may be causing them to swallow excess air. Seeking help from a lactation consultant can ensure your baby is latching correctly.

- **Avoid tight clothing and slumped positions:** Tight clothing around your baby's tummy or slumping in a car seat can exacerbate reflux. Try to keep your baby in a more upright position and avoid slouched postures after feeding.

- **Gentle winding:** Try to avoid vigorously patting or bouncing your baby after a feed, as this may make reflux worse. Instead, gently hold your baby upright on your chest to help relieve any trapped air.

- **Elimination diet:** In some cases, reflux may be linked to food sensitivities, such as a cows' milk protein allergy. Keeping a food diary and eliminating certain foods, like dairy, may help reduce symptoms.

When to Seek Medical Help

If your baby is not gaining weight, is vomiting frequently (as opposed to spitting up) or seems to be in constant distress despite your efforts, it is crucial that you seek medical advice. It is vital that if you notice your baby is showing signs of dehydration, such as fewer wet nappies, or if the reflux is accompanied by fever or blood in their stool, make sure you seek medical attention urgently. They may want to investigate further to rule out other conditions or offer treatment options like medication.

A Word of Reassurance

Reflux is incredibly challenging, but it's important to remember that it's usually just a phase. Babies are incredibly resilient and as their bodies mature and they can sit upright independently, they will gradually outgrow this condition. In the meantime, your responsiveness to their needs – holding them upright, offering shorter, more frequent feeds and giving extra cuddles – will be the best medicine. Know that you are doing an incredible job, even when it feels tough. Each day, you're nurturing and comforting your baby and that bond will be a foundation of strength for you both. Keep trusting yourself, and remember that this stage, as difficult as it may feel right now, is temporary. I don't write this lightly, especially because I appreciate just how exhausted you may be as you read this. But, as difficult as this stage is, I also believe that knowing that it *is* temporary allows you to focus on getting through each day in the knowledge that things really will get better in time.

Until that time, lower your expectations of how each day should look. Set yourself free from preconceived notions of what your days *should* look like and focus instead on what you, your baby and your family need right now. It can be difficult to do this in the throes of the fourth trimester, so here are some questions to guide you through doing so:

1. What do you and your baby *need* today?
2. How do you want to feel by the end of the day?
3. What do you need to do (or not do) in order to feel that way?
4. Who can help with this?

Accepting that this phase is incredibly challenging is not defeatist, it's wise. This simply is not the season for adventurous baby classes. There is plenty of time to teach your baby how to swim. I promise.

Teething and Breastfeeding

Ah, teething – one of the great rites of passage in babyhood. If you've ever experienced it, you'll know that it's not just your baby's gums that are sore. It can bring a whole host of challenges for you too. The thing is, although teething can make nursing uncomfortable for your baby, it can also be the time when breastfeeding becomes more vital than ever. Breast milk contains powerful natural analgesics that can soothe and relieve your baby's sore gums, and many babies instinctively nurse more when they are teething to comfort themselves.

As your little one's gums become swollen and red and their usual pattern of biting or chewing everything in sight escalates, it's entirely natural to worry about whether breastfeeding can continue without becoming a painful experience for you both. In fact, many mothers fear that teething will cause their baby to bite or clamp down on the breast. And while that is a terrifying thought, there are steps you can take to manage the situation with love and patience.

How to Manage Biting During Teething

The first thing to remember is that your baby is not trying to hurt you. It may feel like their new teeth are a tiny set of razors, but their biting is most certainly about their need for comfort than any intention to cause pain. At their tender young age, they have no concept of others' feelings. When your baby bites during breastfeeding, it's often because they're trying to relieve the pressure or discomfort in their gums. Biting whilst nursing can sometimes happen when your baby loses focus or becomes distracted, or when they latch poorly out of frustration.

Here are a few gentle strategies to manage biting:

1. **Stay Calm:** If your baby bites, try to remain calm and avoid screaming or pulling away. Sudden movements might startle them and lead to a nursing strike or make them think that you are playing a game! Instead, gently break their latch by placing your little finger between their gums and your breast to break the seal.

2. **A Deep Latch:** Encourage a deep latch by guiding your baby to open their mouth wide before latching on. The deeper the latch, the less likely your baby is to bite. You can model this to your baby by demonstrating a wide, open mouth yourself.

3. **Provide Comfort:** When your baby is in discomfort, use breastfeeding to soothe their sore gums. If your baby starts biting, offer them something to gnaw on before the feed, such as a clean knotted muslin dipped in breast milk and frozen.

4. **Nipple Care:** If your nipples are sore from breastfeeding or biting, help your body heal by applying some breast milk to the area. Your freshly expressed milk has natural healing properties that no store-bought cream or balm can match. Silver cups are also great for soothing and protecting your nipples during recovery, as they have antimicrobial properties that can promote healing.

   Additionally, nipple shields can sometimes be used to help manage nipple pain, especially if you have nipple damage or if your baby is struggling to latch properly. These silicone shields fit over your nipple and can provide a protective barrier, allowing your nipples to heal while still allowing your baby to feed. However, a word of caution: while nipple shields can be helpful in the short-term, they should not be used as a long-term solution without guidance from a lactation consultant. Overuse can interfere with your baby's latch and milk transfer, potentially leading to other issues like low milk supply or discomfort. Always consult with a professional before using nipple shields to ensure they're the right choice for your situation.

It's important to remember that teething is a phase and while it may bring moments of pain, it doesn't mean the end of your breastfeeding relationship. Keep trusting in your ability to provide comfort and nourishment to your baby during this time.

Nursing Strikes: When Baby Refuses the Breast

A nursing strike is another challenging part of breastfeeding that can happen when your baby who has previously been feeding well suddenly refuses the breast. It can feel devastating, especially if it's unexpected. You may find yourself asking,

'Is this the end of my breastfeeding journey?' The short answer is no, it's not the end, though it can certainly feel that way in the moment.

Nursing strikes often occur when something disrupts your baby's usual feeding routine. While teething can be a big trigger (as sore gums can make feeding uncomfortable), nursing strikes can also happen for a number of other reasons, including illness, stress or even changes in your milk supply. For us, it was a particularly stubborn flu-like virus that left my son congested and unable to nurse because he couldn't breathe at the same time.

> *Tip: if your baby is congested, try nursing them in a steamy bathroom, as the water vapour will help to clear their airways.*

Signs of a Nursing Strike

If your baby suddenly refuses the breast, it can be helpful to first rule out physical discomfort, such as teething pain or congestion. If they seem healthy but are still refusing to latch, they may be experiencing one of the following:

1. **Teething Pain:** If your baby is teething, the pressure from breastfeeding can hurt their gums. They may refuse the breast temporarily, especially if they associate the pain with nursing.

2. **Illness:** Colds, ear infections or other illnesses can make breastfeeding uncomfortable for your baby. They may want to nurse less frequently or not at all during the height of their discomfort.

3. **Overstimulation:** Too much activity or new environments can make babies feel overwhelmed and less

interested in breastfeeding. Sometimes, they'll refuse to nurse due to being overstimulated.

4. **Milk Supply Changes:** If your milk supply has fluctuated, it might have made feeding less satisfying for your baby. This can lead them to reject the breast in favour of a bottle or other methods of feeding.

How to Handle a Nursing Strike

It's important to do all that you can to stay calm and remember that this is likely a temporary phase. Here are some tips to help you through it.

1. **Keep Offering the Breast:** Even if your baby is refusing, continue to offer the breast frequently but in a low-pressure way. Try to choose moments when they are relaxed, such as right after waking or before sleep. Skin-to-skin contact – like taking a bath together – can help your baby feel more secure and may encourage them to latch.

2. **Offer Expressed Milk:** If your baby is refusing the breast entirely, express milk and offer it in a bottle or cup. This ensures they are getting the nourishment they need while you work through the strike. Maintaining your milk supply is vital during this time, so regular expressing (or pumping) is key to avoiding a drop in supply. Aim to express at least as frequently as your baby would normally nurse, ideally every three hours or so during the day. It can feel like a lot, but it's key to keep stimulating your breasts.

3. **Create a Calm, Relaxed Environment:** Try to make feeding time as calm and quiet as possible. Reduce

distractions, dim the lights and hold your baby close to your chest to encourage comfort. The more relaxed the atmosphere, the more likely your baby is to feel secure and open to feeding.

4. **Stay Close and Comfort Your Baby:** Sometimes a baby will refuse the breast because they're going through a phase of increased separation anxiety. Hold your baby close, offer them unrestricted comfort and reassurance with your voice. Remember that your tone of voice and your body language are communication too. Providing emotional comfort during this time is just as important as meeting their physical needs.

5. **Be Gentle and Patient with Yourself:** A nursing strike can be emotional and it's easy to feel frustrated or worried. I'll never forget sobbing in bed as my baby fell asleep in my arms, and my engorged breasts leaked. 'What if that's it?' I asked my partner through bleary eyes. Ask the people around you to care for you and speak kindly to yourself, knowing that you're doing the best you can. You are not alone in this, and your efforts are seen and valued.

6. **Be Mindful of Clogged Ducts:** As you continue to express milk to maintain your supply, be mindful of the possibility of clogged ducts. When milk is not being fully emptied from your breasts, it can lead to blockages which can be painful and, if left untreated, may lead to mastitis. It's important to remember that any lump or hard area in your breast should always be worth investigating with a medical professional. While clogged ducts are common, it's crucial to seek medical advice to rule out other potential causes, especially if the lump persists or is accompanied by other symptoms like fever or redness.

To address a blockage, make sure to massage your breasts gently while expressing, focussing on any areas that feel particularly full or tender. If you notice any hard lumps, you can try applying cool compresses or using gentle massage to encourage milk flow. Regular expression is key – don't forget to continue expressing to help clear any potential blockages. For more detailed information on how to manage and treat clogged ducts, please refer to page 156 where we go more in-depth on this topic.

A nursing strike can be an incredibly confusing time, but remember that it is highly unlikely to last beyond a few days – especially if your baby is under one. Trust that your bond with your baby is still intact. Keep offering comfort and nourishment and trust that with time and patience, your breastfeeding relationship will resume. Take comfort in knowing that you are still providing your baby with love and care – just in a slightly different way for a little while.

> Mantra to Remember: *This is temporary. I trust my baby and I trust myself.*

Breastfeeding and Sleep Disruptions

If you're anything like millions of new mothers around the world, you might think it's your responsibility to teach your baby how to sleep. Yes, sleep is essential, and if your little one is anything like mine, an overtired baby or toddler can be a handful! But you might drive yourself mad if you think it's your job to teach them to go to sleep. This myth is often perpetuated by the multi-million-pound sleep training industry. The truth is, sleep is a biological function, not a skill we can teach. So why, you may wonder, do all of the other parents you know swear by conventional sleep-training methods?

Studies have shown that babies who are 'taught' to sleep using cry-it-out methods do learn one thing: they learn that no one is coming, no matter how long or how hard they cry. As a result, their little bodies go into a kind of learned helplessness, becoming still and silent. While some babies might stop crying and fall asleep quicker than others, the evidence suggests that cortisol (the stress hormone) levels remain high, even after they stop crying for their caregivers. This might make life easier for parents, but it doesn't necessarily help our babies sleep longer or wake up less frequently.

As parents, we do have a role in creating a safe, comforting environment for sleep. But there are times when the white noise is on, the blackout blinds are closed, the room is the perfect temperature and your baby is fed, with a fresh nappy and a full tummy – and they *still* aren't asleep after 90 minutes of back-breaking rocking, patting, shushing and nursing. And you know what? That's okay. Infancy, toddlerhood and early childhood are periods of drastic physiological and psychological change. There will be times when your little one doesn't sleep the way experts say they should. Here are a few possible reasons why:

- A developmental leap (their rapidly growing brains have a lot to process!)

- Teething (more often than you might have anticipated)

- Wind

- Overtiredness

- Under-tiredness

- Sensitivity to stressful situations around them

- Their temperament!

Whatever the reason, please know that it's not your fault that your baby is struggling to sleep. You don't need to sleep-train and you certainly don't have to teach them to 'self-soothe' (newsflash – it's impossible to teach a baby or toddler to do this!). You're not responsible for making your baby sleep in the way society tells us they should.

There may of course be times when illness is preventing them from sleeping, but that's not what I'm referring to here. Give yourself grace if you're feeling at your wits' end. Your child will sleep independently and longer stretches when they're ready – without you doing a single thing to encourage it – just like every other human being in history. In the meantime, here are some tips I found really helpful during those sleepless nights.

1. Acceptance

My number one tip is probably the least popular but most impactful: acceptance. It was the single greatest thing that helped me cope with as little as four hours of broken sleep a night. I don't just mean accepting that your child is awake but accepting that they are not a solid sleeper right now – just like most babies, toddlers and young children around the world. I truly believe that if this fact was acknowledged and discussed more openly and honestly among communities, it would ease so much pressure on new parents.

2. Never Clock Watch

Never, I repeat, *never* look at the clock when your little one wakes up overnight. It won't benefit you, and if you're anything like me, it'll only rob you of more sleep as you watch the minutes tick by wondering if you'll ever get back to sleep before your baby wakes again.

3. **Stay Hydrated**

Hydration makes a huge difference to both your body and mind, especially when you're sleep-deprived. I got into the habit of keeping a pint of water by my bed overnight, ready to drink first thing in the morning. This simple act has helped combat the brain fog that often clouds my mind after a sleepless night.

4. **Forget Household Chores**

Forget about anything non-essential that doesn't contribute to rest and bonding with your baby. If you live with someone, talk to them about how, while you're on night duty, they can help with other responsibilities at home. If you live alone, don't hesitate to ask friends or family for support. Put the pile of laundry out of sight and repeat outfits where possible. If cooking from scratch feels exhausting, ask loved ones to prepare meals for you once a week and forgive yourself for having more sandwiches and ready meals than you'd like. Take a breastfeeding multivitamin and add fresh vegetables and salads wherever possible to make your meals more nutritious.

5. **Rest or Sleep When Baby Sleeps**

If you're able to nap during the day, try to take advantage of those moments. If you can't, aim to go to bed at the same time as your baby each night. Yes, you might miss out on binge-watching your favourite shows, but those extra hours of sleep are invaluable. You might be able to catch an extra sleep cycle, making the next day much more bearable.

6. **Meditate**

Meditation is a restorative practice for tired minds. It's scientifically proven to reduce anxiety and depression during pregnancy and beyond. Personally, I credit meditation with supporting me through the toughest times in my life, including divorce, miscarriage and postpartum anxiety. Whether you've meditated before or not, I encourage you to try a guided sleep meditation to help calm your mind and restore balance.

As part of the Resources section I've created for you (see page 305), I've included a series of guided meditations that can support you through moments of stress, exhaustion and overwhelm. These recordings are designed to be simple, soothing and easy to follow, even if you've never meditated before.

Life on little sleep can feel like you are wading through treacle, but that doesn't mean it can't still be filled with moments of love and joy. While it may seem like this season of sleeplessness will never end, I promise that it will. In the meantime, give yourself permission to surrender to the moment. Be kind to yourself and let go of unnecessary pressures. Set yourself free of the 'shoulds' and don't engage in comparisons with others – as the saying goes, a flower does not think of competing with the flower next to it, it just blooms. So let your little bud do just that.

When I stopped holding myself responsible for my son's sleep, I embraced him as the whole, perfect individual he is – quirks, sleep habits and all. His personality is something I will never try to change, because I adore him exactly as he is.

Yes, it's tough, but I believe that anything worth having comes through hard work. So, breathe with me, mama. Inhale wisdom and strength, exhale the belief that you can control your baby's sleep. When we fully accept our children for who they are, we allow them the space to grow in mind and spirit. And if we do that, can you imagine what the world will be like for them when they grow up? If you ask me, it's a world worth fighting for.

Nipple Thrush

As a mother, you know how overwhelming breastfeeding can feel at times. It can be difficult enough to navigate the challenges of latch, milk supply and sleepless nights without the added concern of pain or discomfort during feeds. When you bring the possibility of thrush into the mix, it can seem like yet another hurdle to overcome.

Thrush, or candidiasis, is a yeast infection caused by an overgrowth of *candida* fungi, which can affect both you and your baby. It is most commonly seen in breastfeeding mothers and can cause a range of uncomfortable symptoms. I have personally experienced nipple thrush twice. On both occasions the infection began as a bright pink, itchy patch on my nipple which burned like a flame when my son nursed. For me it was not toe-curlingly painful as I had heard it being described, but it felt like a sharp, sore pain. A deep, comfortable latch helped me manage the pain until I could get treatment for myself and my son each time.

What Is Thrush?

Thrush can affect the nipples, the inside of your baby's mouth or both. In mothers, it often manifests as sharp, stabbing pain during or after breastfeeding. Nipple thrush is an infection caused by the overgrowth of a yeast called *candida albicans*, which is naturally present in small amounts in the body, including on the skin, in the mouth and in the gut. When there is an overgrowth of this yeast, it can lead to an infection in the nipple area, causing symptoms such as pain, redness and burning sensations during or after breastfeeding.

Signs of Thrush

For mothers, thrush may cause:

- **Sharp, stabbing pain** in the nipple area during or after feeding.

- **Itchy or burning** sensations on the skin of the nipple or areola.

- **Cracked, flaky or scaly skin** on the nipple or redness that doesn't heal.

- **Shiny, red skin** around the nipple area, with or without pain.

- **Painful or tender breasts**, even between feeds.

- **Nipple pain that doesn't improve** with positioning or latch adjustments.

For babies, thrush may cause:

- **White patches** inside the mouth (on the tongue, gums or inside the cheeks) that don't wipe off easily.

- **Fussiness or discomfort** during or after feeds, as the yeast infection can make sucking painful.

- **Difficulty latching** due to the discomfort caused by thrush in their mouth.

- **Nappy rash**, which can be a secondary symptom of thrush if the infection spreads.

Known Causes of Nipple Thrush

1. **Antibiotic Use:** One of the most common causes of thrush is the use of antibiotics, which can disrupt the balance of healthy bacteria in the body, leading to an overgrowth of yeast. This can affect both the mother and the baby. If the mother takes antibiotics for a condition such as mastitis or if the baby is given antibiotics (for example, for an ear infection), it can increase the risk of thrush developing.

2. **Yeast Transfer:** Thrush can be transferred between mother and baby. If the baby has thrush in the mouth (oral thrush), it can be passed back to the mother's nipples during breastfeeding, especially if the baby has a poor latch, is gumming or chewing the nipple or is frequently sucking for comfort.

3. **Cracked or Damaged Nipples:** Any cracks or damage to the skin of the nipple create an opportunity for the yeast to enter and infect the area. Poor latch, improper positioning or ineffective sucking can cause nipple trauma, making the skin more susceptible to infection.

4. **Weak Immune System:** A compromised immune system can make it easier for yeast to overgrow. Conditions like diabetes, a weakened immune system due to illness or medication, or even stress can contribute to this.

5. **Moist or Warm Environment:** Yeast thrives in warm, moist environments. Wearing tight, non-breathable clothing such as synthetic bras can trap moisture and heat, providing an ideal environment for yeast growth. It is also common for thrush to develop when breastfeeding mothers wear nursing pads that are not

changed regularly, as they can become moist from breast milk.

6. **Hormonal Changes:** Hormonal fluctuations, particularly those occurring during pregnancy, menstruation or with the use of hormonal contraceptives, can also make mothers more susceptible to yeast infections.

7. **Other Factors:** Other potential contributing factors to nipple thrush include smoking (which can reduce the body's natural ability to fight infection) and poor hygiene practices, such as not washing the breasts on a regular basis.

Sugar Intake and Nipple Thrush

The link between sugar intake and thrush is related to the way yeast thrives. Yeast feeds on sugar, so when there is an excess of sugar in the diet it can promote the growth of yeast, increasing the risk of thrush.

1. **Increased Sugar Availability:** A diet high in refined sugars, processed foods and carbohydrates can increase blood sugar levels, which in turn can create a more favourable environment for yeast growth. Yeast feeds on sugar and when sugar is abundant in the body, it can encourage the yeast to overgrow leading to an infection like thrush.

2. **Weakened Immune System:** Excessive sugar intake can suppress the immune system, making it harder for the body to fight off infections, including fungal infections like thrush. It is important to maintain a balanced diet that supports the immune system, which includes moderating sugar intake.

3. **Candida Overgrowth:** Candida is naturally present in the gut and its overgrowth is often linked to an imbalance in the gut microbiome caused by high sugar intake. This overgrowth can potentially spread to other parts of the body, including the mouth (causing oral thrush) and the nipples (causing nipple thrush).

Managing Nipple Thrush

1. **Diet and Sugar Reduction:** Reducing refined sugar and processed carbohydrate intake may help prevent the overgrowth of candida. A diet that includes a balance of whole foods, high-fibre vegetables and lean proteins can support the immune system and reduce the likelihood of thrush infections.

2. **Probiotics:** Adding probiotic-rich foods (such as yoghurt, kefir and fermented vegetables) or taking a probiotic supplement can help restore the balance of healthy bacteria in the body, which may prevent yeast overgrowth.

3. **Treatment:** If thrush is suspected, both the mother and the baby may need to be treated with antifungal medication, often in the form of topical creams for the nipples and oral medication for the baby. It's essential to follow the treatment plan prescribed by your healthcare provider to ensure that the infection is cleared up.

4. **Hygiene and Moisture Control:** Keeping the nipple area dry and clean is important. Change nursing pads frequently and wear loose, breathable clothing to reduce the moisture that can fuel yeast growth.

5. **Addressing Latch Issues:** Ensuring that your baby is latching well and your nipples are not damaged is crucial in preventing nipple thrush. Working with a

lactation consultant to correct latch problems can really help too.

How Does Thrush Affect Breastfeeding?

The pain caused by thrush can lead to significant difficulty breastfeeding. For some mothers – myself included – the fear of the pain that comes with each feed may cause them to feel anxious or reluctant to nurse. This can create a stressful cycle of tension and discomfort, not only affecting your physical well-being but also your emotional state as you continue your breastfeeding journey.

It's also worth noting that thrush can be passed between you and your baby. If your baby develops oral thrush, the infection can then be passed back to you through breastfeeding. This means that both of you need to be treated simultaneously to prevent re-infection.

How to Prevent and Treat Thrush

1. **Consult a healthcare professional:** The first step in managing thrush is to get an accurate diagnosis. A doctor or lactation consultant will be able to assess whether thrush is the cause of your discomfort and can provide guidance on appropriate treatment options.

2. **Use antifungal treatments:** If thrush is diagnosed, your healthcare provider may prescribe topical antifungal creams for your nipples and oral antifungal treatments for your baby. It's important to follow the prescribed treatment to ensure that both you and your baby are fully treated and to avoid re-infection. Both of you will typically need to be treated at the same time.

3. **Good hygiene practices:** To prevent the spread of thrush, it's important to practise good hygiene. After

every feed, try to clean your nipples gently with warm water and let them air dry. Wash your hands thoroughly before and after breastfeeding. Be sure to sterilise any items that come into contact with your baby's mouth or your breasts, such as pacifiers, teething toys and breast pump parts.

4. **Avoid scratching or rubbing the area:** If your nipples are cracked or sore, avoid any irritation that might worsen the condition. It can be tempting to try to alleviate the discomfort by rubbing or scratching, but this can make things worse.

5. **Breastfeeding positioning:** Ensure that your baby has a good latch and they're feeding effectively. Poor latch can aggravate nipple pain and make it harder for your nipples to heal. Consider reaching out to a lactation consultant for advice on positioning and latch if you're experiencing ongoing issues.

6. **Switch to breathable fabrics:** Wearing breathable, non-synthetic fabrics can help avoid creating a moist, warm environment, which is ideal for the growth of yeast. Consider wearing cotton bras and tops and avoid tight, non-breathable fabrics.

7. **Supportive self-care:** The pain and frustration that comes with thrush can take an emotional toll. Remember to be kind to yourself during this challenging time. Take breaks when you can, prioritise rest and reach out for support from family, friends or a lactation consultant. Self-compassion is key here.

When to Seek Help

If you're treating thrush and you're not seeing improvements after a few days, or if the pain becomes unbearable, please reach out to your healthcare provider. Sometimes thrush can persist and you may need an alternative treatment. Also, if you notice that your baby's thrush symptoms are not improving or if they develop any secondary issues such as a persistent nappy rash, it's important to follow up for further support.

A Word of Reassurance

I understand how incredibly frustrating and painful thrush can be. It can make a challenging period of breastfeeding even more difficult, but it's important to know that it's something that can be treated and managed. With the right care, you'll be able to overcome this hurdle and continue your breastfeeding journey with more comfort and less stress.

Thrush is temporary, and as difficult as it may feel right now, it won't last forever. You're doing a wonderful job caring for your baby and this is just one of those tough phases that you'll eventually look back on as something you worked through together. Keep trusting yourself and remember: You are capable and this challenge will soon be behind you. Hang on tight, mama.

Clogged Ducts and Mastitis

Mastitis and clogged ducts are two of the most uncomfortable and sometimes distressing challenges in a mother's breastfeeding journey. It's frustrating, painful and at times feels like an overwhelming setback, especially when you've worked so hard to establish a smooth breastfeeding routine. However, as with many facets of motherhood, these hurdles too shall pass – and with the right care and support, you can continue to thrive on your breastfeeding journey.

What Are Clogged Ducts and Mastitis?

A clogged duct occurs when milk gets trapped in one of the tiny ducts in the breast. It may feel like a small, hard lump and can sometimes cause mild discomfort. If left untreated, however, a clogged duct can develop into mastitis – an infection of the breast tissue, often accompanied by pain, redness, swelling and flu-like symptoms, such as fever and chills.

It's important to remember that clogged ducts don't always lead to mastitis, but if you're feeling pain, tenderness or noticing changes in your milk flow, it's crucial to address it as early as possible. Mastitis, if not treated promptly, can become more serious and cause further complications, such as abscesses. But don't be alarmed; these issues can often be managed effectively with the right treatment.

Causes of Clogged Ducts and Mastitis

Clogged ducts typically occur when milk isn't drained properly from the breast. This can happen due to various factors such as a poor latch, engorgement or even wearing tight clothing that puts pressure on your breasts. Sometimes breastfeeding more frequently or nursing on one side can also result in milk not being fully emptied from the breast.

Mastitis usually develops when a clogged duct becomes infected. This infection often happens when bacteria enters the breast tissue through cracked or damaged skin, typically around the nipple. However, sometimes mastitis can occur without an obvious blocked duct, often triggered by rapid milk production or other physical stress on the breast.

Warning Signs

With a clogged duct, you might notice a small, tender lump in your breast that may or may not be accompanied by pain or redness. Sometimes, it may feel like a blockage that's difficult to clear. If the lump remains, it becomes more painful, or if you begin to feel flu-like symptoms such as fever or chills, it may indicate that the blockage has turned into an infection, leading to mastitis.

Mastitis typically presents with swelling, redness, warmth in the affected breast and the flu-like symptoms mentioned above. You might also experience deep, throbbing pain and discomfort that can make it feel impossible to nurse your baby from the affected side.

If you experience any signs of infection, such as fever, redness spreading or severe pain, contact your healthcare provider immediately. Mastitis, if left untreated, can be more serious and may require antibiotics.

How to Manage Clogged Ducts and Mastitis

1. **Keep Breastfeeding:** As hard as it may seem, continuing to breastfeed is one of the most effective ways to relieve a clogged duct and begin the healing process for mastitis. Nurse frequently and offer the affected breast first, as your baby's strong suck can help relieve the blockage. A good latch is crucial here, so consider seeking support from a lactation consultant to ensure your baby is latched on correctly and milk is flowing freely. If nursing on the affected side is too painful, try expressing the milk manually or with a breast pump to relieve the pressure.

2. **Your Milk is Still Good:** Your breast milk isn't infected and it's still perfectly good for your baby, although the taste may change slightly. This is because sodium and chloride levels increase in your milk, which may cause your little one to fuss or even refuse to nurse altogether.

3. **Gentle Massage:** While nursing or pumping, gently massage the affected area. Start from the outside of the breast and move towards the nipple. This can help encourage milk flow and clear the blockage. Be gentle, as too much pressure could cause further discomfort.

4. **Stay Hydrated and Rest:** As with any illness, your body needs hydration and rest to heal. Drink plenty of fluids and try to rest whenever possible. Your body is working hard to fight the infection and clear the blockage, so allow yourself time to heal.

5. **Pain Relief:** If you're experiencing significant discomfort, over-the-counter pain relievers such as paracetamol or ibuprofen can help. The Drugs In Breast Milk Service run by The Breastfeeding Network offers free information and advice from a team of pharmacists.

6. **Seek Medical Help if Needed:** If your symptoms don't improve within 24 hours, or if you develop a high fever, worsening pain or swelling, it's essential to consult your healthcare provider. In some cases, antibiotics may be required to treat mastitis and it's safe to use them while breastfeeding. Your healthcare provider will recommend the most appropriate treatment to support your recovery.

The Emotional Toll

Dealing with the pain of mastitis or clogged ducts can be emotionally draining. As mothers, we often feel the weight of wanting to be perfect and 'do it all' when it comes to our babies. But please remember, experiencing these challenges doesn't mean you've failed, nor does it define your ability to breastfeed. It's okay to feel frustrated, upset or even angry when you're in pain, but it's also important to practise self-compassion. Mastitis is just one of the many hurdles that can arise during your breastfeeding journey, but it is not the end of the road if you don't want it to be. You are resilient and your body is incredibly capable of healing with the right support and care.

Milk Blebs

Milk blebs, also known as milk blisters, are one of those painful but relatively common challenges many breastfeeding mothers face. As a new mother, you may have already experienced the discomfort of a bleb without fully understanding what it is. It's a small, often painful white dot that forms on the nipple or areola.

While milk blebs may not always hurt, when they do the discomfort can be sharp and localised, making breastfeeding or even just touching your breast feel unbearable. Sometimes these blebs can resolve themselves over a few weeks with no treatment at all, but when they're painful or persistent, there are steps you can take to manage the condition.

What Causes Milk Blebs?

Milk blebs are most often the result of blocked milk ducts or inflammation in the breast tissue. They may occur when the milk in a particular duct backs up, causing the duct to become inflamed, with milk eventually blocking the nipple pore. Mastitis can also play a role in the development of milk blebs, as inflammation caused by infection or congestion can lead to a bleb forming at the surface of the nipple.

It's important to understand that while a milk bleb can be frustrating and painful, it's not always a sign of something more serious, although it can sometimes be a surface symptom of underlying inflammation or infection. If the pain is severe and persistent, it's important to keep an eye on any other symptoms, such as fever or increased redness, as these can indicate an infection like mastitis, which may require more intervention.

Can I Continue to Breastfeed with Milk Blebs?

Yes! The good news is that you can continue breastfeeding with a milk bleb. In fact, breastfeeding may help reduce the inflammation in your breast. However, it's important to avoid excessive feeding to clear the bleb, as this can stimulate increased milk production, potentially worsening the inflammation. Instead, feed your baby based on their natural hunger cues. Additionally, it's best to avoid trying to remove the bleb by squeezing or massaging the breast, as these actions are ineffective and can lead to further tissue damage. Gentle, responsive feeding is the most effective approach to manage and resolve a milk bleb.

If you are finding it particularly difficult to nurse with the bleb present or if the pain is unbearable, there are ways to manage it more effectively.

Tips for Managing Milk Blebs

Here are a few things you can do to alleviate the discomfort and help heal the bleb.

1. **Apply Cold to the Affected Area:** Use a cold compress or an ice pack wrapped in a cloth to reduce the inflammation in the tissue behind the bleb. This can help soothe the area and ease the pain.

2. **Soak the Nipple in Warm Water:** A warm soak or compress after breastfeeding can help soften the skin and promote better milk flow. You can gently massage the area during the soak to encourage the milk to move more freely and possibly help the bleb clear.

3. **Wear Cotton Soaked in Olive Oil:** Some mothers find relief by wearing a cotton ball soaked in olive oil inside their bra. This can help soften the skin, providing some comfort and possibly promoting healing.

4. **Avoid Squeezing or Picking at the Bleb:** As tempting as it might be, do not try to pop the bleb yourself. While you might feel temporary relief from releasing the milk, doing so can lead to infection, more inflammation or the bleb reforming. It's always better to let a healthcare professional manage this if the bleb doesn't resolve on its own.

5. **Keep Breastfeeding Frequently:** Even if breastfeeding is uncomfortable, it is one of the most effective ways to clear the bleb. Frequent feeds will help to relieve pressure in the breast and encourage milk flow through the duct.

6. **Pain Relief:** If the pain is becoming overwhelming, you may find that taking over-the-counter pain relief like paracetamol or ibuprofen helps. This will not only manage the pain but also reduce inflammation, allowing the skin to heal more comfortably.

7. **Ask About Medication:** If these at-home remedies aren't providing relief, you can consult your healthcare provider about using a steroidal cream to reduce inflammation and allow for better milk flow. Some women also find relief from taking over-the-counter lecithin or choline supplements, which help thin the milk and can prevent further blockages.

When to Seek Professional Help

In most cases, milk blebs will heal on their own with time and proper self-care. However, if you're experiencing severe pain or the bleb doesn't clear up with the steps mentioned above, it's time to seek professional help. A lactation consultant or your healthcare provider can assess the bleb and may recommend de-roofing it with a sterile needle to relieve the blockage. This is typically a safe procedure when done by a professional, but it's essential to continue breastfeeding afterwards to prevent the bleb from reforming.

Embracing Patience and Self-care

Having a milk bleb can be frustrating, but it's important to be kind to yourself during this time. Remember, this too shall pass. Your body is working hard to keep your milk supply flowing and to nurture your baby. Sometimes obstacles like milk blebs are simply part of the journey. Approach this challenge with patience, knowing that it's just a temporary phase.

Take care of your body by staying hydrated, eating well and asking for help when needed. Give yourself permission to rest and allow your body the time it needs to heal. Keep in mind that your breastfeeding journey is about connection, nourishment and providing your baby with what they need. This includes recognising when to pause, seek support and give yourself the grace to move through the challenges with compassion.

Raynaud's Syndrome and Nipple Blanching

If you've experienced sharp, shooting pain in your nipples or noticed that your nipples change colour after a feed, you may be dealing with something called Raynaud's Syndrome or nipple blanching. While the two terms are often used interchangeably, there's a subtle difference between the two. But don't worry, either way, the good news is that you're not alone and there are steps you can take to relieve the discomfort and make breastfeeding more manageable.

What is Raynaud's Syndrome and Nipple Blanching?

Raynaud's Syndrome is a condition where the blood vessels, particularly in the fingers or nipples, constrict in response to cold or stress. This can cause the affected area to become pale or white and can lead to pain when the blood flow returns. When it occurs in the nipples, it can cause them to blanch (turn white), then they may turn a bluish or purple colour and eventually return to normal as blood flow returns. The sharp pain can feel like a sudden, intense burning or stinging sensation.

Nipple blanching, on the other hand, is a term used more generally to describe the loss of colour in the nipple area during or after breastfeeding. This can happen without the intensity of pain that accompanies Raynaud's but can still be uncomfortable or alarming.

Why Does This Happen?

For many mothers, the sudden discomfort or colour changes in their nipples after breastfeeding can feel bewildering, but it's important to remember that this is not a reflection of your ability to nurse. As one client remarked, 'It was like my son sucked all the life and colour out of my nipples at every feed!' Raynaud's Syndrome in the nipple area is often related to temperature changes or the physical response to breastfeeding itself. When the baby latches, the pressure applied to the nipple can sometimes cause temporary constriction of blood vessels, and if the weather is cold, or if there are sudden shifts in temperature (e.g. moving from a warm room to the cold air outside), this can trigger the response.

For some mothers, stress or fatigue can also play a role in this constriction, especially if you've been dealing with breastfeeding difficulties or sleep deprivation. The body's stress response can affect blood flow and, in turn, cause these symptoms to appear.

Signs and Symptoms

The signs of Raynaud's Syndrome or nipple blanching typically include:

- **Pain:** A sharp, burning or stinging sensation in the nipple, often occurring during or after feeding.

- **Colour changes:** Your nipple may turn white, pale or even bluish, followed by a return to its usual colour once blood flow is restored.

- **Cold or numbness:** Some women experience a sensation of coldness or numbness in the nipple area, which can be particularly noticeable if exposed to a drop in temperature.

Managing Your Symptoms

The first thing to remember is that while these symptoms are uncomfortable, they are usually temporary and can be managed with a bit of care and attention.

1. **Keep Warm:** One of the simplest ways to prevent Raynaud's and nipple blanching is to stay warm. Keeping your body, especially your chest, warm during feeds can help prevent the blood vessels in your nipples constricting. Wearing warm clothing, including a soft nursing bra or breast pads, can help protect your body from temperature fluctuations.

2. **Use Heat Before and After Feeds:** Applying a warm compress or warm water to your breasts before a feed can help promote better circulation and reduce the likelihood of Raynaud's. After nursing, you can also try massaging your breasts gently to encourage blood flow back to the area.

3. **Gentle Latching:** A good latch is crucial not just for comfort, but also for maintaining healthy circulation. A shallow latch can increase pressure on the nipple, leading to further constriction. Ensure your baby is latched deeply, with their mouth covering both the nipple and a good portion of the areola. If you need help with latch issues, don't hesitate to reach out to a lactation consultant or a breastfeeding support group.

4. **Switch Positions:** Experiment with different nursing positions to see if one helps alleviate the pain and pressure in your nipples. Sometimes, changing the angle or how your baby latches can help reduce symptoms.

5. **Breastfeeding-friendly Clothing:** Be mindful of tight clothing, bras or nipple shields that could put pressure on your nipples or affect blood circulation. Opt for loose, comfortable clothing that doesn't restrict blood flow.

6. **Reduce Stress:** As with many breastfeeding challenges, stress can exacerbate symptoms of Raynaud's. Try to rest, breathe deeply and reduce sources of stress as much as possible. Your emotional well-being is just as important as your physical health.

7. **Consider Supplements:** Some mothers find that supplements, such as lecithin or choline (a supplement that can help improve milk flow and reduce the risk of clogged ducts), may also help manage symptoms. It's

worth discussing with your healthcare provider whether this is a good option for you.

8. **Consult a Healthcare Provider:** If the pain becomes too much or the symptoms don't improve, it's important to speak with a healthcare professional. They may recommend further treatments, such as topical medications or, in more severe cases, prescription options like vasodilators, which can help improve blood flow.

It's completely understandable if you're feeling frustrated or worried by these painful symptoms, but remember, you're doing so much, all of the time. As always, be kind to yourself and know that these symptoms are often temporary. Your body is working hard to care for your baby and sometimes it just needs a little extra attention to keep everything flowing smoothly. Moments like these are a part of your beautifully imperfect journey. If you need additional help, don't hesitate to reach out to a lactation consultant, support group or your healthcare provider.

Breastfeeding Aversion and Agitation (BAA)

Breastfeeding is often portrayed as a beautiful, natural bonding experience between mother and baby. However, for many mothers the reality can be far more complex and challenging. One such challenge is Breastfeeding Aversion and Agitation (BAA), a phenomenon that remains under-researched despite impacting a significant number of breastfeeding mothers. If you find yourself grappling with intense negative emotions while breastfeeding, know that it's not just you, mama.

What is it?

Breastfeeding Aversion and Agitation (BAA) is a phenomenon where you might experience particular negative feelings and intrusive thoughts when your baby is latched and suckling at the breast. These emotions can include anger, irritation, disgust and even rage, often accompanied by physical sensations such as itching or a 'skin crawling' sensation. These feelings are unexpected and almost always unwanted, as many mothers experiencing BAA would like to continue breastfeeding.

For instance, you might find yourself having an overwhelming urge to de-latch your baby, only to be overcome with guilt and confusion afterwards. The distressing emotions usually disappear once the baby stops breastfeeding, but the impact on your mental and emotional well-being can be significant.

My Experience

I first encountered BAA when my son was approaching his third birthday. It caught me completely off guard, as I had previously loved nursing him on demand and felt like it was a huge privilege to be able to do so. Seemingly out of the blue, I started to feel frustrated and found myself nursing him through gritted teeth. What was going on? Was I finally ready to stop nursing? I felt consumed with guilt, as my son was still very much attached to breastfeeding and I had hoped to allow him to self-wean. In the end, I couldn't continue. I didn't want my memories of breastfeeding to be dominated by negative emotions. If this is the case for you too, you can read about deciding whether or not you should continue breastfeeding in Chapter Ten (see page 265).

> ### Distinguishing BAA from Dysphoric Milk Ejection Reflex (D-MER)
>
> It's important to differentiate BAA from another condition, called Dysphoric Milk Ejection Reflex (D-MER). While both involve negative emotions during breastfeeding, they are distinct phenomena. D-MER is characterised by feelings of dysphoria, such as sadness or anxiety, that occur with the release of milk (your let-down) and typically dissipate shortly afterwards. In contrast, BAA involves persistent feelings of anger or agitation throughout the feeding session, which only subside once the baby, toddler or child stops suckling.

Common Triggers and Experiences

BAA can be triggered by various factors, including hormonal changes, pain during breastfeeding and physical sensations caused by your baby's behaviour, such as nipple twiddling, biting or fidgeting. You might also find that BAA is more prevalent when you're tired or during your menstrual cycle, indicating a possible link to hormonal fluctuations.

Many mothers describe feeling 'touched out' or overwhelmed by constant physical contact, especially those who are tandem feeding or breastfeeding demanding toddlers. This sensation of being overwhelmed can exacerbate the negative emotions associated with BAA.

The Emotional Toll

The emotional toll of BAA is profound. Like me, you might struggle with intense feelings of shame and guilt, torn between the desire to nurture your child and the intense aversion you feel during breastfeeding. This internal conflict can lead to distress and a sense of failure, as you try to reconcile your negative emotions with societal expectations of joyful breastfeeding.

While there is limited research, there are some strategies that might help you manage these difficult emotions. Cognitive distraction techniques, such as focussing on something else during breastfeeding, taking certain supplements and seeking support from other mothers who understand what you're going through can be beneficial. Speak to your doctor about getting your vitamin and mineral levels checked to see if supplementation might be required to help you feel better. It's also crucial (though rarely easy), to prioritise self-care, ensure you are well-rested and maintain a balanced diet to help mitigate some of the triggers for BAA. If this feels impossible, read my tried-and-tested, no-nonsense approach to long-term breastfeeding self-care at the end of Chapter Five (see page 204).

Seeking Support

If you're experiencing BAA, D-MER or any other challenges on your breastfeeding journey, reaching out for support is essential. Online support groups can provide a sense of community and understanding, helping you see that you are not alone in this struggle. Sharing your experiences with healthcare professionals, a lactation consultant, supportive friends or fellow breastfeeding mothers can also provide you with additional resources and support tailored to your needs. There is strength in sharing your experiences and knowing you're not alone. Yes, breastfeeding can be incredibly hard at times, but it's also the best thing I have ever done in my life. If you feel that way too, know that your nursing and pumping journey is worth fighting for, irrespective of any bumps in the road.

In this chapter, we've explored the many challenges that can arise during your breastfeeding journey, from hormonal changes and oral ties to colic and reflux. We've discussed practical strategies for dealing with common obstacles like nursing strikes, clogged ducts and teething and I hope you now feel empowered with the tools and knowledge to navigate these hurdles with confidence.

It's important to remember that these hurdles are all part of the process and, with the right support, they can become stepping stones towards a deeper connection with your baby. The journey of breastfeeding isn't always easy, but it is full of powerful moments of growth, love and connection. Keep nurturing yourself, trusting in your body's ability to adapt and heal and remember that every obstacle you face is one you can overcome with the right support.

In the next chapter, we will dive into the essential practice of self-care, exploring how you can nurture your own well-being amidst the demands of breastfeeding. Caring for yourself is just as crucial as caring for your baby, and in this next chapter you'll find practical tips and compassionate guidance to help you prioritise your health, both physical and emotional, so you can keep showing up for yourself and your little one.

CHAPTER FIVE

Nurturing Yourself

One of the greatest challenges of self-care as a nursing or pumping mother today is the stark reality that, for many, we aren't being taken care of in the way we truly need. Whether it's because of economic pressures, where our partners or families are working hard to make ends meet and physically cannot take on the caregiving role, or because of societal expectations that place the burden solely on mothers, the reality is that self-care often becomes an afterthought. In modern life, many of us are left to navigate this complex, demanding role of motherhood on our own, without the communal support that once was a staple of family and village life. This leaves many of us in a position where our own needs are overlooked.

Finding Strength Within

Since becoming a mother and having the immense privilege of helping mothers around the world through my work, I've come to realise that we don't have to rely solely on society or others to take care of ourselves. While it's lovely to be cared for, there are times when our circumstances don't allow for that – and in those moments I've learned that we are not powerless. And neither are you, mama. In fact, it was breastfeeding that showed me that I can nurture myself as I care for my son because, guess what? There are no greater lovers and carers on Earth than us mothers. So, what if we lavished some of that abundant love and adoration on ourselves too?

It probably took me around four and a half years after the birth of my son to finally put into practice the loving care I give myself with as much devotion as I dote on my incredible child. Sharing this deeply wholesome and, for me, life-changing wisdom feels like a piece of magic that I have been entrusted to share with you. Breastfeeding is actually the perfect analogy for maternal self-love and self-care because lactation offers myriad protective benefits for mothers just as it does for our babies. I realised this on a quiet Sunday morning around 5am, when my son, unwell, nursed on and off in the early hours. I was so grateful that I didn't have to physically get out of bed and pace around the room with him between feeds – my partner did so to comfort him – because it didn't have to be him or me – it gets to be both of us.

Recognising the Demands

While systemic change is essential – such as better lactation support and equitable maternity leave – the reality is that, in the short-term, we need to take care of ourselves as best we can. And I don't think there is anyone better than us to decide what that looks like.

Exhaustion and depletion are often a real part of our breastfeeding experience, especially in those early months. It can feel overwhelming at times. Yet, in a society where breastfeeding is often seen as a privilege – something to be celebrated – many mothers end up feeling alone and drained by the constant demands. We don't often talk about the toll breastfeeding takes on mothers, nor do we discuss the full picture of breastfeeding as a physical, emotional and mental endeavour that requires deep care, both from others and from ourselves.

This is where breastfeeding self-care becomes so very vital. It is an essential practice that needs to be prioritised as an integral part of life as a nursing and pumping mother. While breastfeeding is indeed a privilege in the sense that not all mothers can do it, it's equally true that it is incredibly demanding. Taking care of yourself is not just about treating yourself to occasional indulgences or small self-care practices. It's about recognising the full extent of what your body is doing for your baby and honouring those needs. Your physical, mental and emotional energy are all deeply tied to your ability to nurture your child.

Self-care isn't just about adding more to your to-do list. It's about carving out space, acknowledging your needs and respecting your body's demands as it works tirelessly to nourish the one you love most.

It is my absolute honour to guide you through how to care for yourself as you nurture your child in this chapter. Together, we'll explore how to balance your needs with the demands of motherhood and how to embrace self-care as an essential and nourishing practice – one that is as vital as the care you give to your baby.

Understanding How Breastfeeding Affects You

Before you can understand how to take care of yourself as a nursing or pumping mother, you need to understand how lactation affects you – beyond the size of your boobs! Breastfeeding is a deeply transformative experience that profoundly affects how we as mothers think, feel and engage with ourselves and our families. The act of nourishing your baby with your body connects you to the primal, magical rhythms of motherhood while simultaneously demanding an extraordinary amount of physical, emotional and mental energy. This section delves into the ways breastfeeding influences mothers, offering you the context to better understand how to care for your own wellness during this precious yet challenging time.

The Psychological and Emotional Effects of Breastfeeding

Breastfeeding influences you in myriad ways, shaping your mood, stress responses and even how we interact with others. On a physiological level, it triggers the release of oxytocin, which not only facilitates milk let-down, but also fosters feelings of calm and bonding. Research has shown that breastfeeding mothers often report lower levels of stress, anxiety and negative mood compared to formula-feeding mothers.

This isn't just perception – it's backed by physiological changes. Breastfeeding mothers exhibit stronger cardiac vagal tone, which refers to the activity of the vagus nerve in regulating heart rate and promoting a calm, balanced state. A higher cardiac vagal tone is associated with emotional resilience, meaning your body is better equipped to handle stress. In addition to this, breastfeeding mothers show lower blood pressure and reduced heart rate reactivity, indicating a calmer, less anxious state which I remember vividly to this day. Furthermore, breastfeeding mothers tend to have a reduced cortisol (stress hormone) response to social stress, suggesting that breastfeeding provides a natural buffer against the emotional turbulence of early motherhood.

What does this mean for you? It means that breastfeeding can be a source of emotional stability, helping you feel more connected to your baby and better equipped to handle the ups and downs of parenting. However, it's also important to acknowledge that every mother's experience is unique – if you're feeling overwhelmed, anxious or low despite breastfeeding, it doesn't mean you're doing anything wrong.

The Magic of Mother–Infant Attachment

One of the most enchanting aspects of breastfeeding is its role in fostering attachment between mother and baby. Feeding at the breast is an act of intimacy and connection. The skin-to-skin contact and physical proximity create a space where your bond can truly flourish. Research has shown that breastfeeding mothers are more likely to touch their infants, respond sensitively to their cues and spend time in mutual gaze. These interactions lay the foundation for secure attachment, building a relationship rooted in trust and love.

On a neurological level, breastfeeding activates emotional brain regions, enhancing your sensitivity to your baby's needs. For example, functional MRI studies reveal that breastfeeding mothers show heightened brain responses to their baby's cries compared to formula-feeding mothers. These changes are thought to help mothers become more attuned to their infants, strengthening their relationship.

However, it's worth noting that breastfeeding is just one pathway to a secure attachment. While it can facilitate bonding, attachment is ultimately built through the loving care you provide in *all* areas of your baby's life. Whether you're breastfeeding, bottle-feeding or using a combination of both, the most important factor is the love and attention you bring to your interactions.

Breastfeeding and Postnatal Depression (PND)

The relationship between breastfeeding and PND is complex. Many studies suggest that breastfeeding is linked to lower rates of PND, with mothers who breastfeed for longer durations reporting fewer depressive symptoms. Oxytocin plays a role here – its calming and mood-enhancing effects may help protect against feelings of sadness or overwhelm.

Yet, difficulties with breastfeeding can sometimes contribute to depression, especially if challenges like low supply, pain or latch issues lead to early cessation. For some mothers, the emotional weight of wanting to breastfeed but struggling to do so can be significant. This underscores the importance of seeking help and addressing challenges early, whether through lactation support, counselling or simply talking with a trusted friend or family member.

It's also vital to remember that your mental health is just as important as your baby's physical health. If breastfeeding is causing you distress or exacerbating existing mental health challenges, it's okay to reassess your feeding choices. You are no less of a mother if you make decisions that prioritise your emotional well-being over any particular way of feeding your baby. On the contrary, that makes you a hero.

Understanding Your Constraints and Freedoms

Self-care as a breastfeeding mother is not about striving for perfection – it's about honouring your own needs alongside your baby's. Rest when you can. Eat nourishing foods. Lean on your support network. Give yourself grace in moments of struggle and celebrate your incredible capacity to nurture. Here, we'll dive into the practical steps that you can take to look after yourself as a nursing or pumping mother, armed with the knowledge that you deserve unique attention and care at this particular time of your life.

Mindfulness and Breathwork

One of the most powerful mindset shifts you can make is to recognise that not every action in your day needs to revolve exclusively around your baby 24/7. While it's natural to want to meet their needs with your full attention, it's equally important to understand that taking care of yourself doesn't take away from your ability to be there for your child. In fact, it enhances your ability to nurture them when you make time to care for your own well-being.

This may sound simple, but for many of us – myself included – it's a mindset shift that requires (a lot of!) practice. It's easy to feel that every moment must be dedicated to your baby, especially when the demands of motherhood feel endless. But what if you allowed yourself to believe that nurturing yourself is just as important as nurturing your baby? It is not a choice between your well-being and theirs – actually, the more you care for yourself, the better you can care for them.

For example, when your baby is feeding, instead of feeling you must be constantly on high alert, try using those moments to rest your body and mind. Take a moment to check in with yourself and take a few deep breaths.

Incorporating mindful breathing into your breastfeeding routine is a form of somatic breathwork. Somatic breathwork uses intentional breathing patterns to bring awareness and healing to the body. You can find more information about these techniques in Chapter One (see page 37). By taking deep, slow breaths, you activate your parasympathetic nervous system – the part of your body responsible for relaxation. This shift from stress to calm helps you feel grounded, more present and better equipped to connect with your baby in those precious moments of nursing. Breathwork, alongside other somatic practices, can be incredibly powerful tools for parenting.

Grounding is a technique that helps us reconnect with the present moment and our physical bodies. It's a practice of being mindful of your surroundings and the sensations in your body – whether it's the feeling of your feet on the ground or the touch of your baby's skin against yours. These moments of pause, though brief, allow us to reset and create some space between ourselves and the constant demands of motherhood.

> ### Finding Calm through Grounding Practice
>
> A simple yet meaningful grounding practice during breastfeeding could be focussing on your baby's fingers and toes as they nurse. As you count them, you bring your awareness back to the tactile and precious details of the moment. By zoning in on these small, loving sensations, you're fostering a deeper connection with your baby while also calming your own nervous system. This grounding practice helps to anchor you in the present, nurturing your bond while creating a peaceful space for both you and your little one.

By bringing intentional breathwork and grounding into your daily routine, especially during nursing, you're allowing yourself to nurture both your body and your mind. These moments of stillness allow you to recharge, recalibrate and, most importantly, be more attuned to your baby's needs. The beauty of these practices is that they don't require you to step away from your baby – rather, you can use them to enhance your connection while also taking care of yourself. As you ground yourself in the present, you become better able to respond to your baby with patience, love and a calm sense of presence.

It can feel hard to let go of the idea that you always have to be doing something for your child – whether that's feeding, comforting or attending to every cry. But even in the most devoted forms of attachment parenting, it's essential to recognise that your emotional and physical energy is limited, and it's important to step back and acknowledge that your needs matter too.

You don't have to take grand actions to care for yourself every day – small, simple acts can make a meaningful impact. Maybe it's going to bed a bit earlier to get a restful night's sleep, or perhaps it's asking a friend or family member to help out with the baby so you can take a few moments to do something you enjoy, even if it's just for ten minutes. It could be as simple as sitting quietly when your baby naps, soaking in the silence or allowing yourself to take a bath without feeling rushed.

There will be times when your child's needs feel urgent, and that's okay too. Motherhood is not about perfection or achieving some impossible balance every single moment. It's about flexibility and learning to meet your child's needs alongside your own. If you've ever thought, 'I just need a break,' you are not alone. And giving yourself permission to step away, even if just for a short time, is an act of self-love which will ultimately help you to continue being the loving, patient and present mother you want to be.

Making Time for Yourself

When you're in the trenches of new motherhood, it's crucial to protect the precious moments you can carve out for yourself just as fiercely as you protect your baby. In the early days of breastfeeding and pumping, this often requires support from your partner, family or friends. If that support is available to you, delegate some tasks – like cleaning up at the end of the day – so you can preserve a small window of time for rest and relaxation.

If that support isn't available, consider simplifying tasks where possible. For example, opting for paper cups and plates can help avoid the cleanup routine after meals. Even just once a week, allow someone else to handle the tidying up and plan to use that time to recharge.

If you have older children, involve them in helping around the house. Turn tidying up into a fun bedtime game, like 'collecting treasure' from the floor. No, your three-year-old won't tidy up as efficiently as you, but they will still make a difference and that's one less task for you. By allowing them to help, you're also teaching them the value of contributing to the household, while freeing yourself to spend those precious 30–60 minutes after bedtime actually resting, instead of diving straight into chores.

Learn to prioritise 'me-time' with just as much enthusiasm as you plan activities for everyone else. How can you create sacred and protected time, free from other obligations as much as possible? Consider what that would look like and see what small steps you could take to make this happen.

Modelling Self-care for the Next Generation

One of the reasons why so many modern mothers struggle to prioritise and practise self-care, especially in the early days of nursing and pumping, is that we have not seen others do the same. In many ways this has become a generational pattern. As mothers, we are often the first to step up and give and the last to rest, because that's what we've been taught or witnessed from those around us. It's ingrained in us to put our children's needs above our own, but what happens when we don't care for ourselves?

By prioritising self-care, you're not only giving yourself the physical and emotional space you need, but you're modelling to your children that mothers need and deserve time for themselves – and this is the way we can create generational change.

This ties into a psychological concept known as the *internal working model*. The internal working model refers to the mental framework or map we develop in childhood, based on our early experiences with our caregivers. It shapes how we view ourselves, others and the world around us, as well as how we approach relationships. Essentially, our first relationships with our caregivers serve as a template for future relationships, including how we care for ourselves and others. For example, if a child observes their parents taking care of themselves – whether by setting healthy boundaries, relaxing or seeking help when needed – they learn that self-care is an important part of life.

By modelling self-care, we are teaching our children, even if they are too young to understand the specifics, that it's okay to make time for yourself. This lesson is far-reaching. It teaches them to value their own needs, respect their boundaries and understand that caring for others should not come at the expense of caring for themselves. This mindset becomes ingrained in them, becoming part of their own internal working model. When they grow older, they will carry this understanding into their own relationships.

Journal Prompts

Ultimately, the importance of self-care extends beyond the individual and has a lasting impact on how future generations will care for themselves and each other. By making self-care a priority now, we are creating a healthier, more sustainable approach to family life – one that values rest, reflection and the understanding that our needs are just as important as anyone else's. Here are some journal prompts to help you do just that:

Note: These prompts are designed to help you explore the concept of self-care by guiding you to reflect upon your beliefs, childhood experiences and the legacy that you want to create for your family. Be kind with yourself as you work through them – taking or leaving those that do not serve you. Do not hesitate to seek professional mental health support if you need to do so. You can find a list of mental health support services around the world on page 305.

1. **When was the last time you truly prioritised your own well-being?** What did that look like?

2. **How do you feel about the idea of taking time for yourself?** What emotions come up when you think about stepping back for self-care?

3. **Who first taught you that caring for yourself was secondary to caring for others?** How has this belief shaped your actions and choices as a mother?

4. **Think of a time when you felt 'touched out' or overwhelmed.** How could you have responded to that feeling with more compassion for yourself?

5. **What do you need to feel nurtured and cared for right now?** What small steps can you take today to meet those needs?

6. **If you were to model self-care for your child(ren), what would that look like?** What would you want them to learn from your actions?

7. **What messages about self-care did you receive growing up?** How are those messages influencing the way you care for yourself as a mother?

8. **How would you describe your relationship with rest?** Do you feel you deserve it? Why, or why not?

9. **How can you begin to say 'no' with more confidence?** What would it look like to protect your time and energy in a way that nurtures you?

10. **Imagine your child(ren) coming to you in the future, asking how they should take care of themselves.** What advice would you give them about balancing their needs with the needs of others?

11. **What is the one thing you've been neglecting in your life because you're focussed on your children's needs?** How can you begin to nurture that part of you again?

12. **Think about a moment when you felt guilty for taking time for yourself.** What would you say to another mother who feels the same guilt?

13. **How does caring for yourself benefit your family?** In what ways does your own well-being ripple out and impact your relationships with your children and partner?

14. **What would your life look like if you believed that taking care of yourself was just as important as taking care of your child(ren)?** What steps can you take to make this belief a reality?

15. **Who do you admire for how they take care of themselves?** What do you think they've understood about self-care that you may still be learning?

The Power of Music

Music has the remarkable ability to transform your mood and nurture your well-being, especially during the postpartum period when you may be feeling physically and emotionally drained.

Instead of constantly playing 'The Wheels on the Bus' or your child's favourite lullabies on repeat, try putting on *your* favourite tunes as well. Think of how music reminds you of times before motherhood, when you had much more space for your own tastes and needs – what does that feel like, to be transported momentarily? This isn't about drowning out your baby's cries or avoiding your child's needs; it's about gently merging the pre-mama version of you with your mother edition.

Beyond just listening to music, consider moving with it too. Dancing with your baby can be a wonderful, free way to bond while giving your body a little movement. Whether you're swaying in a rocking chair or dancing around the living room, it's a beautiful way to engage both of you in a nurturing experience, help keep your energy up and remind your body that you too need movement and rhythm, just as your baby does. These moments, while simple, can work wonders for both your mental and physical well-being. The family dance-parties established in those lonely lockdown months remain a precious, firm fixture in our home to this day.

If your baby, like mine, is particularly sensitive to noise, you can start with the music at a lower volume and invest in a good set of earphones for yourself – nothing too fancy – but just enough to create a peaceful escape when you need it. These small efforts to bring a little piece of joy, sound and movement into your day can recharge your spirit, helping you stay grounded and centred in the often chaotic rhythm of new motherhood.

The Magic of Nature

Nature has an incredible ability to heal and restore and even just a brief moment spent outdoors can offer profound benefits for both you and your baby. It's something that is often spoken about in the world of wellness, but in the haze of new motherhood, it can seem like a daunting task. How do you find the time or energy to step outside with a toddler and a newborn who refuses to be put down for more than 30 seconds? The answer is: slowly and without pressure.

Depending on your circumstances, it may not be realistic to get outside every day, and that's alright. Many of the mothers I work with find that getting out for a brisk walk once or twice a week feels more achievable. If it's not possible to shower beforehand or get everything done before heading out, don't worry about it. Sometimes, just putting one foot in front of the other is enough.

If it serves you and feels right, consider stepping outside for a walk with your baby in a sling or stroller. If you're able to, try to aim for a natural setting, like a park, garden or wooded area, as the grounding effects of nature will be even more profound. If it's safe to do so, you might even kick your shoes off and spend some time grounding by walking (mindfully) on the bare earth or grass, barefoot. Even if it's just for 10–15 minutes, being outside in the fresh air and natural surroundings can be an instant mood booster. Those small moments of connection with nature – whether you're basking in sunlight or listening to the rain fall – can help you feel more centred and rejuvenated, even on the toughest days when you're running on little sleep.

Hydration: The Foundation of Wellness

Taking care of your body begins with hydration and proper nutrition, especially when you're breastfeeding. Your body works hard to nourish your baby and keeping yourself hydrated is essential for maintaining your energy and well-being. Breastfeeding burns up to 500 calories a day and your body needs more fluids to replenish what's being used. Water is crucial for milk production as breast milk is approximately 90 per cent water. The more hydrated you are, the better you'll feel and the more effectively your body can produce milk.

A simple yet effective strategy is to drink a glass of water every time you sit down to nurse. It helps you stay on top of hydration and can prevent headaches, which were all too common in the early days of breastfeeding. Keep a large glass or bottle by your bed and drink it as soon as you wake up in the morning. This small habit will help you hydrate consistently, even on those sleep-deprived foggy days.

Breastfeeding and Alcohol

Alcohol can have a negative impact on our mood, health and overall quality of sleep, and even more so when you are nursing or pumping. The NHS advises nursing mothers that, 'An occasional drink is unlikely to harm your baby, especially if you wait at least two hours after having a drink before feeding . . . Regularly drinking above the recommended limits can be harmful for you and your baby.' The American Academy of Pediatrics provides similar guidance, adding that alcohol can impact milk production.

These recommendations are based on the fact that it takes around two hours after consuming alcohol for your blood alcohol levels to return to zero as a breastfeeding mother. If you choose to consume alcohol while breastfeeding, it's important to know that your blood alcohol levels peak around 30–60 minutes after drinking, or 60–90 minutes after if consumed with food. Therefore, if you want to minimise the amount of alcohol passed on to your nursling through your milk, it's best to feed either as you are drinking or several hours after you've had a drink.

Does Alcohol Pass into My Milk?

In short, yes, alcohol does pass into your milk in tiny quantities. However, it's important to know that alcohol passes into and out of your milk freely as your body metabolises it.

Therefore, there is no need to pump and dump simply because you've had a glass of bubbles at a party. But if you've consumed large amounts of alcohol, it's advisable to wait a few hours until your blood alcohol levels have decreased before nursing or pumping.

While the amount of alcohol in your breast milk may be your primary concern as a nursing or pumping mother, it should not be the only consideration. For instance, if you choose to consume alcohol while breastfeeding, it's important to remember that you should not bedshare with your baby after drinking. Additionally, after consuming multiple alcoholic drinks, you might feel tipsy or even drunk. In this state, your ability to care for your baby could be compromised due to the risks of falling or other safety concerns. While it may be safe for you to nurse your little one after drinking, caring for them safely could be the greater challenge. With this in mind, it's advisable to plan for another loving caregiver to look after your child after a particularly merry night out.

How Might My Child Be Affected?

We've established that if you consume alcohol as a breastfeeding mother, tiny amounts will pass on to your baby if you nurse them within around two hours of having a drink. But how might even small amounts of alcohol affect your baby? This will depend on several factors, including:

- The age of your baby or child.
- The amount of alcohol consumed.
- The frequency with which alcohol is consumed.

Younger babies are more readily affected by alcohol consumption than toddlers. Regularly consuming large quantities of alcohol will also have a greater impact on your nursing child than the occasional drink or two. Some known effects of regular, excessive alcohol consumption on breastfed babies include:

- Nursing less frequently and consuming lower volumes of milk.
- Decreased time spent in active sleep.
- Negative effects on cognitive development and abilities.

For these reasons, regularly consuming large quantities of alcohol is not recommended for breastfeeding mothers at any stage of their nursing or pumping journey.

How Does Alcohol Affect Breastfeeding?

Alcohol use can also influence breastfeeding in several ways that you should be aware of. These include:

- A temporary decrease in milk production.
- Inhibition of the milk-ejection (let-down) reflex.

Consequently, excessive alcohol use has been shown to contribute to a decrease in the overall duration of breastfeeding, meaning the number of weeks or months that mothers continue to breastfeed their babies.

The side effects mentioned above have been observed in nursing mothers who have consumed excessive amounts of alcohol or have done so over prolonged periods. Drinking the occasional glass of fizz on a special occasion is generally considered safe, even when nursing your baby on demand. If you feel apprehensive about feeding your baby breast milk that contains even tiny amounts of alcohol, simply wait a few hours before doing so. Whether breastfeeding or not, if you ever feel as though you are relying on alcohol for your mental health or as a coping mechanism, please seek support from your GP or Health Visitor sooner rather than later. Despite what our culture often portrays, you do not have to rely on alcohol to get through the day and if you do, you deserve help to find less-maladaptive coping mechanisms.

Baby-wearing: The Freedom to Move

For new, nursing and pumping mothers, rest is essential. Your body has just gone through an immense transformation and it's important to honour your need for healing and recovery. Baby-wearing can be an incredible tool, but it should never be seen as a way to hyper-productively manage every task during the early days with your newborn. In fact, during this time, your body still needs ample rest and nurturing. It's okay to let things slide a little and take the time to simply rest with your baby, whether that means lying down, sitting together or even taking a nap.

That being said, if you find yourself in situations where your baby absolutely refuses to be put down and you need to get things done, baby-wearing can be a beautiful solution. It's a way to keep your baby close, secure and comforted, while allowing you to move around the house or even venture outside for a walk. Whether you're trying to make a meal, tidy up or simply take a moment to breathe while doing small tasks, baby-wearing offers a chance to gently balance the demands of motherhood with your own well-being.

Baby-wearing is not a new concept; it's been a part of caregiving traditions in many cultures around the world for centuries. In many communities, it's not only a practical solution, but also a deeply-rooted cultural practice. For example, my partner's side of the family is Zimbabwean and baby-wearing is a staple part of their culture. In Zimbabwe, babies are traditionally worn on the back, wrapped securely with a cloth around the caregiver's chest and waist, held in place with a series of tucks and rolls. As someone who is half Zimbabwean,

I knew that my son would instinctively love being worn with pride on my back, just as the women in my family had done for generations.

However, when I first tried baby-wearing, it didn't go as smoothly as I had imagined. My son wasn't as fond of the back carry as I had hoped. At first, I assumed I just didn't have the technique right. With some advice from his grandmother and some practice, I refined my method – but even then, my son wasn't as keen to be on my back as I had expected. He loved being close to me, he just wanted access to my boobs 24/7 too.

It was then that a thoughtful gift from my sister – a fabric sling – came into play. This simple piece of cloth was exactly what I needed. Unlike the more structured carriers, the sling offered flexibility and comfort. My son, being a 'boob monster' through and through, took to it right away. With practice, some trips to the local sling library and a few trial runs before I mastered the art of walking and nursing at the same time, I eventually found a new lease of freedom. Once my son was nestled against me, I was able to move around, get some fresh air and regain a little bit of independence.

Baby-wearing Care and Caution

It is essential to remember that baby-wearing can be dangerous if not done safely. Improper positioning can lead to suffocation, particularly for newborns or premature babies whose airways are more fragile. This is why seeking professional advice before you start baby-wearing is crucial. Consulting with a baby-wearing expert or a trained sling consultant can ensure that you are using the right carrier for your baby and that they are positioned safely. Many consultants offer online consultations or can direct you to local sling libraries for hands-on guidance.

Baby-wearing, whether on the front, back or side, is an absolute lifeline for mothers and babies alike. It promotes essential skin-to-skin contact, which is incredibly beneficial for infants as they rely on their caregivers for coregulation of their bodies. This bonding time is crucial for their emotional development. At the same time, it allows mothers to regain some mobility while keeping their babies close and secure. It was a simple yet powerful way for me to feel a sense of freedom and get a break from the confines of sitting on the sofa or being tethered to one spot all day.

Tag-team Like a Pro: The Power of Shared Responsibility

If you have a partner or a supportive family member nearby, tag-teaming can be a game-changer in preserving your energy and well-being. The early months of motherhood can feel all-consuming, especially when you're navigating the challenges of breastfeeding, sleep deprivation and recovery. But when you embrace the power of shared responsibility, it can make all the difference in ensuring you stay grounded and well.

Tag-teaming doesn't just mean taking turns feeding, although that's certainly helpful. It's about a mutual commitment to supporting each other in whatever way feels necessary. This might mean alternating night shifts for feeding, where your partner takes over while you get a stretch of sleep, or it could involve simply being together with you *and* your baby or children, assisting with the day-to-day challenges of motherhood. For example, your partner might help with bath time, nappy changes or offer a comforting presence while your baby settles for the night. Even when you're breastfeeding exclusively, there are countless ways your partner or a trusted family member can contribute – whether it's prepping meals, doing the laundry or taking over bedtime routines.

Tag-teaming isn't necessarily about someone else taking your child away for long stretches of time (although there's nothing wrong with wanting and needing time away from your children, as long as they are with a loving and responsive caregiver). Often, it's about sharing the load, being present together and offering support in the tasks that make up daily life as a mother of young children.

It's easy to feel like you have to do it all on your own, especially when your baby is so small and dependent. But remember, your partner or loved ones want to help – but they need to know how. Being open about your needs, even if it's as simple as asking for a bit of time to yourself, can strengthen your bond and help you feel more supported. This was certainly my experience, and it is also true of every mother I've worked with one-on-one. You don't have to do this alone.

If the idea of asking for help feels intimidating or overwhelming, start small. You don't have to ask for a whole day of respite, especially when your baby is tiny and breastfeeding is constant. Instead, try carving out 20–30 minutes of uninterrupted time for yourself each day. It might be as simple as taking a quick shower, stepping outside for a walk around the block or going on a solo trip to the grocery store. These small moments of self-care can work wonders for your mental health, giving you a chance to reset and recharge. Think of them as supporting beams, strengthening the bridge of your matrescence.

It's important to remember that taking time for yourself doesn't diminish your role as a mother; it enhances it. When you feel supported and have the space to care for your own well-being, you become a more patient, present and compassionate parent. Just like in any partnership, the more you share the load, the more you're able to fully show up for each other – and for your baby. And when both partners are equally involved, it sets the tone for a beautiful, balanced relationship where the well-being of everyone is valued and nurtured.

Epsom Salt Baths: A Simple Escape

Epsom salts are renowned for their ability to promote relaxation, reduce stress and provide relief from anxiety. As a new mother, you may often feel like your body is constantly in a state of tension, whether from the physical demands of breastfeeding, the strain of sleepless nights or the emotional intensity of caring for your little one. A bath with Epsom salts can help release some of that tension, providing much-needed respite for both your body and mind.

The magnesium in Epsom salts is absorbed through the skin and is believed to help boost serotonin levels, which can lift your mood and promote a sense of calm. This is particularly important during the postpartum period, when hormonal fluctuations and sleep deprivation can leave you feeling overwhelmed and exhausted. Epsom salt baths can also help soothe sore muscles – whether from nursing, holding your baby or perhaps being on your feet all day. It's a simple and affordable way to nurture your body when you need it the most.

If you are able to indulge in a full bath, take this opportunity to create a little escape for yourself. Dim the lights, light a candle and put on some calming music or simply enjoy the stillness. The warm water will relax your muscles and the Epsom salts will do the rest. Let your thoughts wander and take this time for yourself without guilt. It's a reminder that taking care of you is just as important as caring for your baby.

Stretch and Move: Embracing Gentle Movement and the Wisdom of Yoga

Your body has gone through a significant, permanently life-changing transformation. Now, as you care for your baby, it's important to be kind to yourself, acknowledging the need for physical movement that nurtures and doesn't punish your body. Stretching and gentle movement are powerful ways to care for your body during the postpartum period, especially when you may be spending hours sitting and nursing.

While it's easy to feel the pressure to 'snap back' to your pre-pregnancy body, this is not the goal of postpartum movement. It's about listening to your body, restoring balance and giving yourself the time and space to heal. Gentle stretching, light yoga or even simple movements can be incredibly restorative, without the need for intense workouts or unrealistic expectations.

The Benefits of Stretching and Light Movement

Gentle movement, such as stretching or simple yoga poses, can help release tension that builds up during long hours of sitting while nursing or tending to your baby. When you're breastfeeding, you may find yourself hunching over or sitting for extended periods, which can lead to discomfort in the neck, shoulders and back. Incorporating small stretches into your day can help ease this physical strain, promote circulation and help you feel more grounded and at ease.

Stretching is not just for your muscles – it also provides mental clarity and emotional support. Research has shown that gentle movement can reduce physical discomfort, improve posture and even alleviate symptoms of postpartum depression. Light stretching and mindful movement bring you into the present moment, helping you release stress and reconnect with your body.

Understanding Relaxin: Why Stretching Matters Postnatally

After childbirth, your body is still in a state of adjustment and one reason why stretching and gentle movement are so beneficial is because of the hormone relaxin. Relaxin helps your body prepare for labour by loosening ligaments and joints, particularly in the pelvic region. However, relaxin can remain in your system postpartum, especially if you are breastfeeding. This increased flexibility can make you more prone to muscle strain, so stretching becomes even more important during this time.

Because your ligaments and joints are more flexible postpartum, it's important to approach movement gently and mindfully. You may need to take extra care when exercising to avoid overstretching, as your body is still recovering and adapting.

The Eight Limbs of Yoga: A Holistic Approach to Self-care

Yoga isn't just about stretching and movement – it's a philosophy that guides us towards greater peace, presence and self-awareness. The Eight Limbs of Yoga, a framework laid out in the ancient yogic texts, offer a beautiful, holistic approach to self-care that can be especially beneficial for postpartum mothers. Whether you were quite literally a marathon runner before you fell pregnant or more of a couch-to-5k kind of gal, here's a look at the eight limbs and how they can support you during this transformative time:

1. **Ethical Disciplines: Yama** The first limb of yoga is about how we interact with the world around us. During the postpartum period, this can involve setting boundaries and practising kindness towards yourself. For instance, acknowledging that you deserve time for self-care even when your baby's needs seem endless, is an example of applying the yama of non-violence (*ahimsa*) towards yourself.

2. **Personal Disciplines: Niyama** This limb encourages us to focus on our personal growth and inner development.

Practising contentment (*santosha*) can help you accept your current stage of life as a mother. It's a gentle reminder that this season of motherhood, with all its messiness and exhaustion, is temporary – and that you really are doing wonderfully.

3. **Physical Postures: Asana** This is the part of yoga most people are familiar with – postures designed to improve flexibility, strength and balance. In the postpartum period, your asanas may look different than they did pre-pregnancy, but they are still incredibly important for restoring energy and relieving tension. Think of stretches and gentle yoga poses as a way to tune into your body and ease discomfort. Please take care not to practise even gentle yoga before you have been given the all-clear to do so by a medical professional.

4. **Breathing Techniques: Pranayama** Conscious breathing can help calm the nervous system, reduce stress and restore mental clarity. Incorporating pranayama practices such as deep belly breathing, 4-7-8 breathing or alternate nostril breathing can bring calm and focus to your day, especially during moments of stress or overwhelm. Turn to Chapter One for more guidance on the practice of yogic breathing techniques (see page 37).

5. **Withdrawal of the Senses: Pratyahara** This limb focuses on turning inwards and limiting distractions. It's easy to get lost in the constant external demands of motherhood, but creating moments of quiet for yourself – whether through meditation, a mindful walk or even a few minutes of sitting in silence – can help you reconnect with your inner peace.

6. **Concentration: Dharana** Practising concentration helps quiet the mind and focus on the present moment. In the postpartum period, this could mean focussing on the

simple, tactile experiences of motherhood – like the feel of your baby's skin during a nursing session or tuning in to the rhythm of your breath as you stretch.

7. **Meditation: Dhyana** Meditation is the practice of sustained attention and mindfulness. Even five minutes of meditation can help you feel more grounded and present in your day. Meditation allows you to process the emotional and physical challenges of new motherhood with clarity and compassion.

8. **Enlightenment: Samadhi** The final limb is about achieving a deep sense of connection, peace and oneness. This is about finding balance and peace in your role as a mother. When you practise the other limbs, they naturally guide you towards a greater sense of calm and wholeness. I cannot claim for a moment to have achieved enlightenment! But, motherhood has certainly given me insights into myself which I may never have realised otherwise.

Caring for Your Breasts and Your Milk Supply

Taking care of your breasts and milk production is an essential part of self-care, and it's one of the most important aspects of breastfeeding that should not be overlooked. Your breasts are working hard to provide nourishment for your baby and ensuring that they're comfortable, healthy and well-supported is vital for your own well-being. Wearing a comfortable, well-fitting bra (if you choose to wear one) is a simple yet important way to help prevent discomfort and potential issues such as clogged ducts or mastitis. A bra that fits properly can make a world of difference in terms of comfort, as it helps distribute the weight of your breasts evenly, preventing unnecessary pressure or chafing. Ideally, your bra should provide support without being too tight or restrictive, especially in the early postpartum days when your body is still adjusting to changes in milk production. If you can, use a professional bra-fitting service to ensure the best possible fit.

It's important to be mindful of your body and if you notice any discomfort, soreness, or signs of issues like engorgement or leaks, don't ignore them. Addressing these concerns promptly is not just about relieving discomfort – it's about protecting your milk supply and your overall health. If you're feeling consistently uncomfortable, it's always a good idea to consult a lactation consultant or healthcare professional in person. They can offer guidance on techniques such as breast massage, adjusting your latch or using supportive tools or products, as well as provide support with issues like nipple pain or blocked ducts. Turn to Chapter Four for more guidance on navigating challenges such as these (see page 123).

Taking care of your breasts isn't just about physical comfort – it's also about honouring your body and acknowledging the hard work it's doing. While nursing and pumping are important tasks, they can sometimes take a toll on your body if you're not proactive in caring for yourself. Small acts, such as applying soothing nipple creams or oils, taking warm baths to relax and ensuring you're in a comfortable position while feeding all add up and support your well-being.

If you're dealing with leaks – another common issue – don't feel discouraged. It's completely normal and many mothers experience them, especially in the early days. Try to keeping some nursing pads on hand to protect your clothes or using a breast milk collector to catch any excess milk. Embrace the fact that this is just part of your body's natural process as it adjusts to breastfeeding. If leaks or discomfort are making it difficult to go about your day, don't hesitate to take a moment to relieve yourself. You deserve to feel comfortable and at ease.

Coping with Unsolicited Advice

Dealing with unsupportive comments and unsolicited advice while breastfeeding is one of the most challenging aspects for many mothers. Although breastfeeding is protected by law in the UK, US, Australia and many other parts of the world, nursing in public remains a rarity, particularly when it comes to breastfeeding toddlers or older children. In many Western societies, breastfeeding in front of others can invite unwanted questions, criticisms and scrutiny, even from well-meaning friends and relatives.

Whether you prefer to breastfeed discreetly or more openly, the reality is that breastfeeding can often come with a side serving of unsolicited opinions. So, what can you do about it? Here are some compassionate and effective ways to navigate unsupportive comments with understanding and confidence.

Respond with Facts

Sometimes the best way to manage unsolicited advice is by offering well-researched information. It's empowering to have a few facts in your back pocket when someone questions your choices, or even just to have knowledge of them yourself. Here are some key points you might find helpful:

- Breast milk provides at least 60 per cent of a baby and toddler's vitamin C requirements.

- The immune-boosting properties of breast milk actually *increase* during the second year of life.

- Endorphins in breast milk provide natural, drug-free pain relief when babies and toddlers are teething or unwell.

- Breastfeeding reduces a mother's risk of developing breast cancer by 4.3 per cent for each year that she lactates.

- Studies show breastfeeding is associated with 20–30 per cent increased white matter growth in the brain compared to those who were not breastfed.

- Breastfeeding antibodies have been found in breast milk up to ten months after COVID-19 infection.

These facts can be reassuring and provide clarity when you find yourself under pressure to justify your breastfeeding choices.

Respond with a Sense of Humour

Sometimes, the best way to deflect unsolicited advice is with humour. It can diffuse tension, lighten the mood and turn a potentially awkward situation into something more manageable. It's a way to assert yourself without confrontation, all while giving your body, your choices and your journey the respect they deserve. Plus, who doesn't appreciate a little laugh amid the parenting chaos?

Here are some humorous lines that you can use to deal with well-meaning but intrusive comments:

- 'Excuse me – are you talking about my boobs?'
  This can be a playful way to let the other person know that what they're saying feels a little too personal – and, let's face it, it's a bit awkward to talk about someone's boobs in public.

- 'Are you *still* married to him?'
  For those who ask – 'Are you still breastfeeding?' A cheeky way to turn the focus back on them. If they've got opinions on your personal life, it might be fun to gently remind them that they too have their own relationships to manage.

- 'Are you really going to have another biscuit?'
  When someone comments on your feeding choices or

habits, throw the question back at them. It's a light-hearted way to say, 'We all have our little indulgences, don't we?'

- 'Oh, are we talking about everyone's boobs today? Let's start with yours!'
  This is a cheeky, bold way to deflect the comment and put the spotlight back on them. It's a humorous challenge that can get a laugh while also shifting the conversation.

Humour, when used thoughtfully, can help you navigate tricky situations without escalating things. Just remember, humour is about making things light – not belittling anyone, but making your boundaries clear in a playful and non-confrontational way. By using humour in moments like these, you can stay grounded and confident in your choices while keeping things fun and light!

Respond with Questions

Sometimes, offering questions in response to unsolicited advice can open up meaningful dialogue and help others better understand your perspective. It may also bring insight into why people hold certain beliefs about breastfeeding. Try asking:

- 'What is your experience of breastfeeding?'
- 'What is that opinion based on?'
- 'Why do you feel that way?'

More often than not, answers to these questions reveal genuine curiosity, past trauma, or simply a lack of understanding. I think it's also important to acknowledge that some people can feel uncomfortable around a family member or friend breastfeeding, simply because they're not used to seeing it. This discomfort can stem from personal beliefs, societal norms, or just unfamiliarity with the process. In these cases it's not about the act of breastfeeding itself, but about a general unease that may be rooted in their own experiences or cultural context.

Understanding this discomfort can help foster more open and honest conversations, allowing us to approach the topic of breastfeeding with empathy and patience, rather than judgment.

Respond with Boundaries

As you grow more confident in your motherhood journey, setting clear boundaries becomes easier. It's important to remember that you do not owe anyone an explanation about how you feed your child. Boundaries help you define yourself as both a mother and an individual, allowing you to protect your peace. Here are some boundary setting phrases that may be useful:

- 'I'm really passionate about breastfeeding on my own terms.'
- 'I'm not looking for advice right now.'
- 'Breastfeeding is between me and my baby.'
- 'I love breastfeeding on demand, and it's an active choice I've made.'

You are always entitled to draw the line at comments that feel disrespectful or uncalled for. Your body, your choice and your breastfeeding journey deserve to be respected.

Respond with Compassion

Responding to criticism with compassion can be incredibly healing, especially when the source of the comment comes from someone close to you. For example, many of my closest female relatives have never had the experience of breastfeeding, which has led to insensitive or even hurtful comments at times. If you find yourself struggling with a relative's well-meaning but frustrating advice, try to step back and consider their perspective. Perhaps your cousin, for instance, had a traumatic postpartum experience that left her feeling disconnected from breastfeeding and her insistence that you try formula to help your baby sleep might come from a place of concern, not judgment. Having said that, no-one's experiences or misguided concern gives them the right to think it is appropriate to dictate how you mother or what you do with your own breasts. If necessary, your unsolicited advisor may benefit from a reminder that your breasts aren't up for discussion any more than theirs are.

Most people's opinions about breastfeeding are based on outdated beliefs or generations of misinformation. These views often reflect the lack of support and education available in their time, not a reflection of your choices as a mother. While this understanding might not stop unsolicited comments from happening, it can help you feel less personally affected by them.

Self-care in Action

Remember, you are doing incredible work as a mother. By taking steps to care for your own health and well-being, you're ensuring that you're physically and emotionally equipped to continue giving your best to your baby. Self-care isn't selfish – it's an essential part of being the best, most present version of yourself for your little one.

By practising self-compassion, nurturing your body and seeking support when needed, you are honouring both your needs and the beautiful journey of motherhood. Keep in mind that there is no one-size-fits-all approach – what works for you may look different from what works for someone else, and that's okay. The most important thing is that you're caring for yourself in a way that allows you to thrive as a mother and as a person. You deserve it, and your baby will benefit from seeing you prioritise your own well-being.

CHAPTER SIX

Fuelling Your Breastfeeding

Breastfeeding places unique demands on a mother's body – not just in terms of time and energy, but also in the nutrients required to produce milk, support recovery and maintain overall health. While breastfeeding remains one of the most nutritious options for your baby, it's essential to recognise that your own nutritional health matters just as much during this time. Your body requires an abundance of calories, vitamins and minerals to produce milk and to keep up with the increased physical demands. The importance of fuelling your body with nutrient-dense foods cannot be overstated, as it helps to maintain energy, promote healing and support optimal milk production.

We know that breastfeeding burns up to 500 calories per day, meaning that breastfeeding mothers may need to consume an additional 450–500 calories per day to meet these energy demands. This is no small feat! A nursing or pumping mother is giving so much to her baby, and it's important that she replenish her own resources so that she can keep giving her best.

Various studies have shown that breastfeeding remains the best option for babies, even when a mother's diet is less than perfect. Breast milk continues to provide essential nutrients for your baby even when a mother's nutrition is suboptimal. However, if your diet is consistently missing key nutrients, it's your own body that will bear the cost.

For example, if you don't consume enough protein, your body will pull it from your muscle mass to ensure that your breast milk is nourished. Similarly, if your diet is lacking in vitamin A, your body will take it from your liver to fortify your milk. In the case of zinc, your body will deplete your bones to ensure there's enough for your milk production. When you don't consume enough DHA (omega-3 and Omega-6 fatty acids), your body will pull it from your brain to provide these crucial fats for breast milk. The same goes for calcium – without enough in your diet, your body will take it from your bones to maintain your milk supply.

In addition to these nutrients, your body will also pull from its stores of vitamin C, vitamin D, choline, iodine and B12 if you're not consuming enough of these vital nutrients. As a result, your milk can be lower in these nutrients, which may impact both your own health and your baby's long-term development. I share this information not to make you feel guilty for your far-from-perfect diet, but to highlight why it matters that you are well-nourished and taken care of as a nursing or pumping mama. Your body is working around the clock to provide for both you and your baby. As such, you need help and support to prioritise your health, so that you and your little one can thrive through breastfeeding.

Balanced Diet Tips for Breastfeeding Mothers

In those fragile first days and weeks postpartum, I was lucky to have the support of my Zimbabwean in-laws, who understood the importance of nourishing, home-cooked food during this life stage. They brought mountains of food to our home, and while I was overwhelmed by their generosity, I soon realised that there was much more to it. In many collectivist cultures, there's a deep understanding that new parents need not only emotional support but also practical, hands-on help – especially when it comes to nourishing the body. I remember wondering why we didn't live closer to my fiancé's cousins, aunts and uncles after that first wave of meal deliveries.

If your friends or family are not aware of your need for support, please make them aware. Reach out to someone you trust and ask them to organise a meal train with your friends or community – whether it's through a place of worship or with your child-free friends who may be more than happy to step in. These small, practical supports can make all the difference. As a new mother, you might not always have the energy to prepare balanced meals every day and that's okay. Nourishing your body, however, is non-negotiable.

Snack Stations: Keeping Nourishment Close By

As we touched upon in Chapter Four, I highly recommend keeping snacks nearby – at all times. As you well know, breastfeeding can leave you ravenous and it's easy to forget to eat when you're busy caring for your baby. Healthy snacks such as granola bars, dried fruits, nuts and even hummus (which can be eaten with one hand) are perfect to have on hand. If you can, ask your partner or a family member to help you prepare and stock these snacks. It can make a huge difference, especially during late-night feedings when you're too tired to make a full meal.

Nutrient-rich Meal Planning: Invest in Yourself

If possible, plan your meals ahead of time before your baby arrives. This could mean preparing and freezing meals in advance so that you have easy-to-reheat options once your baby is here. Alternatively, you might budget for a meal delivery service tailored to new parents. Either option is a great way to ensure you have nourishing meals ready during those first few weeks when time and energy are limited. Planning ahead can help take the pressure off and allow you to focus on bonding with your baby instead of worrying about what to cook.

Even if you only manage to plan a few meals, it can relieve some of the pressure when your energy is low. Even better, if you can delegate meal planning or preparation to your partner or other family members, do it! They'll likely be more than happy to help, and it's vital that you prioritise your self-care during this time. If you don't have others in your household, reach out to friends or family nearby. A communal meal plan, where you trade off cooking for each other, can ease the burden on you all.

Batch Cooking

When possible, batch cooking is another helpful strategy. If you or your loved ones can do this before your baby arrives, you'll be set for the busy postpartum period. In fact, I highly recommend that if you can, you buy a chest freezer to fill with homemade meals before you give birth. If you didn't get the chance to batch cook ahead of time, consider making extra portions whenever you do get to cook. Freeze them for those days when you're simply too tired or too busy with your little one to think about cooking. This approach also gives you the chance to nourish yourself with homemade, nutrient-rich meals instead of relying on takeaways or ready-made meals.

By investing a little time in preparing nourishing meals or delegating the task, you ensure that your body is well-fuelled for the demands of breastfeeding. The goal here is not to be perfect but to take small, consistent steps towards prioritising your health. Your body, your baby and your emotional well-being depend on it. And remember, you deserve to be nourished as much as you nourish your child. Don't hesitate to ask for the help you need – you are not alone and support can come in many forms.

Quick and Easy Meal Ideas

Time is precious when you're a new mother and meal prep often takes a back seat. But you don't have to sacrifice your health or your baby's nutrition for convenience. The good news is that there are plenty of quick and nutritious meals you can make, even on your busiest days.

- **Overnight Oats:** Pre-make a jar with oats, chia seeds, pumpkin seeds, your choice of milk and fruit for a nutritious, no-cook breakfast.

- **Smoothies:** Blend fruits, greens and healthy fats (like peanut butter or avocado) and protein for an easy-to-consume meal packed with nutrients.

- **One-pan Meals:** Cook a protein like chicken or salmon with vegetables, all on a single baking tray for easy cleanup and a healthy meal.

- **Snack Boxes:** Keep a container in the fridge with hard-boiled eggs, wholegrain crackers, nuts and fruit for an easy, balanced snack that requires no cooking.

With these simple ideas you can nourish your body and avoid the temptation of processed or takeaway foods, which may be easy to lay your hands on, but are less nourishing.

Let Go of Perfectionism

As with perfectionism in general, this is much easier said than done. However, I will never forget overhearing a fellow mother at a local café. She had a young baby on her lap and was meeting friends. 'I'm starving,' she said, 'We only had sugary cereal bars at home and I'd rather eat nothing than start my day like that.' My heart sank hearing how she had denied herself any sustenance because she did not deem the food that she had at home to be good enough. I've been there, home alone with a hungry baby waiting for a food delivery. But I want you to know that, particularly when you're lactating, any food is better than nothing. That doesn't mean you should live off biscuits, but it's okay if breakfast consists of a handful of mixed nuts, a piece of fruit or some simple toast. Nourishment is key and sometimes, just making sure you get something into your body is enough for the moment.

Foods to Prioritise and Avoid

Anecdotally, foods that *may* support milk production include: oats, leafy greens, garlic, almonds and fennel. Many of these foods can be easily added to your meals – perhaps add a spoonful of ground flaxseeds to your morning oats or snack on a handful of almonds between nursing sessions.

There are other foods to be mindful of: caffeine and alcohol, which can affect milk production and may even alter your baby's sleep patterns – you can learn more about the impact of alcohol on lactation in Chapter Five (see page 187). Moderation with caffeine is key, especially in the early months when your baby's sleep patterns may already be unpredictable. If you're concerned about how these foods affect your milk or baby, consult a lactation consultant, a nutritionist or your family doctor for tailored advice.

In Chapter Four, I talked about how vital choline is for preventing clogged ducts and ensuring that your milk flows well (see page 162). Vegan mothers in particular can be susceptible to having low levels of choline, as they may struggle to consume enough of this nutrient each day without being conscious of their increased need for it. Sources of choline include dairy products, meat, eggs as well as non-dairy sources like soybeans and cruciferous vegetables such as broccoli and Brussels sprouts.

Hydration for Milk Supply

It's easy to become dehydrated, especially in the early days of breastfeeding when you're juggling so much. Aside from drinking water, water-rich foods like cucumbers, watermelon and broths are a great way to supplement your daily fluid intake. Staying hydrated will not only support milk production but also help you avoid the fatigue and headaches that often accompany dehydration. Remember, staying hydrated is one of the simplest yet most effective ways to support your milk supply and overall well-being.

Maintaining Your Energy Levels

Maintaining energy throughout the day is a challenge for many breastfeeding mothers. Your body is working hard to produce milk and take care of your baby, which can leave you feeling drained.

To maintain your energy, focus on eating complex carbohydrates such as wholegrain bread, brown rice, quinoa and sweet potatoes that provide a slow and steady release of energy. Protein-rich foods like beans, nuts and eggs can also help fuel your body. Snacking wisely is also impactful. Choose snacks that combine protein, fibre and healthy fats –a handful of nuts, yoghurt with seeds or avocado toast – to help prevent energy crashes.

How to Manage Food Cravings

Cravings are a natural part of breastfeeding, often driven by fluctuating hormones and the increased energy demands of producing milk. Your body is working hard and it makes sense that you may find yourself reaching for quick sources of energy. Rather than thinking of cravings as something to resist, consider them gentle signals from your body about what it needs. The goal isn't restriction but balance – choosing foods that help sustain your energy rather than leading to highs and crashes.

If you're craving something sweet, try pairing fruit with a source of healthy fat or protein (like nut butter or yoghurt) to keep your blood sugar steady. If you're in the mood for something salty, opt for nutrient-rich options like roast potatoes with a drizzle of olive oil or crunchy roasted chickpeas. And, of course, enjoy your favourite treats mindfully and without guilt – because nourishment is about both joy and well-being. By listening to your body and choosing foods that energise rather than deplete you, you'll feel more balanced, sustained and ready to meet the demands of motherhood.

Nourishing Yourself While Breastfeeding

Breastfeeding is an incredible act of love and dedication and it places unique demands on your body. Your nutritional needs increase, not just to sustain your milk supply but to maintain your own health and energy levels. This chapter has explored how fuelling your body with nutrient-dense foods can help prevent exhaustion, support your milk production and ensure that your own reserves aren't depleted in the process.

We also discussed practical strategies – from meal planning and batch cooking to keeping snacks within easy reach – to help you stay nourished even when life feels overwhelming. And let's not forget cravings! Rather than fighting them, we can reframe them as signals from the body, guiding us towards balance and sustainable energy.

But above all, let's throw perfection out the window. Some days you'll eat a wonderfully balanced, home-cooked meal. Other days, you'll grab whatever is within arm's reach – and that's okay. The goal isn't to stress over every bite, but aim to nourish yourself as much as you nourish your baby. You deserve to feel strong, energised and supported by the food and drinks that you consume.

Now that we've thought about how to take care of your body, let's shift our focus to another vital part of your postpartum experience: your relationships. From your partner to your friends, family and even society at large, breastfeeding can impact the way you connect with others – sometimes in unexpected ways. In the next chapter, we'll explore how breastfeeding weaves into your relationships, how to navigate differing opinions and, most importantly, how to ensure that *you* feel emotionally supported along the way.

CHAPTER SEVEN

Breastfeeding and Your Relationships

Becoming a mother brings about a dramatic shift in priorities and dynamics across all relationships, not just with your partner but also with family and friends. The demands of breastfeeding and pumping affect every aspect of your life. If you have a romantic partner, then this relationship will almost certainly be affected. The transition from being a couple focussed on each other to caring for a new human around the clock can strain even the most solid relationships. This chapter will explore how breastfeeding impacts intimacy, how partners can maintain connection and how to navigate the evolving dynamics of your relationships with friends, family and any romantic partner(s). We will address the challenges that arise with honesty and without judgment, so that your relationships can thrive well beyond your breastfeeding journey.

Your Romantic Relationship

When a baby enters the picture, the focus naturally shifts to their needs – feeding, sleeping and constant care. This is not a slight on either partner; it's simply a fact of life. Babies require 24/7 care and attention because they are completely dependent on others to meet their every need. A key aspect of raising young children that we often overlook in the UK is that this level of care remains essential for at least the first three to five years of each child's life.

While the transition to parenthood is a beautiful one, it can also create tension in your relationship – particularly if breastfeeding is the primary source of nourishment for your baby. Perhaps you used to spend Friday nights at the cinema or watching Netflix and falling asleep in one another's arms. Maybe Saturdays were spent hiking or cruising cafés or beer gardens with friends. Did Sundays used to mean long, lazy lie-ins and time with friends and family? If so, then you and your partner likely had ample opportunity to reconnect after a busy work week. Even if you were both shift workers pre-parenthood, without many other obligatory demands on your time, you would undoubtedly have had space to nurture your love for one another. But with parenthood, those precious moments all but disappear. And if you are breastfeeding, the distribution of care for your baby cannot be equally split, because you spend so much time either nursing or pumping.

In modern society, where breastfeeding rates are among the lowest in the world, many new parents are ill-prepared for the realities of sleep deprivation, cluster feeding and the overwhelming demands of caring for a newborn. It's impossible to fully prepare for the toll that breastfeeding can take on your relationship. The lack of sleep, the constant physical closeness of breastfeeding and the emotional exhaustion that often accompanies this period can create tension and strain.

While you can't entirely predict how breastfeeding will affect your relationship, understanding what is normal – such as frequent night wakings, cluster feeding (nursing for hours at a time) and a new mother's emotional and physical needs – can help you navigate these changes. Knowing that this is a natural part of early parenthood provides reassurance that you're not alone in your experiences. More importantly, this knowledge empowers you to communicate with each other about your realities, your wants and your needs. As a couple, it's vital to check in regularly, acknowledge the challenges and remind each other that you are in this together. If you have a romantic partner, ask them to read and consider the following:

> Imagine that you are about to undergo a procedure which will leave you with a wound the size of a dinner plate, that will heal gradually over around six weeks. During your recovery time, you will be woken up every two to three hours, including through the night. There will be some nights when you will have to stay awake for hours at a time, all while you are healing. Once your physical wound has healed, the night waking may continue for an undefined period of 6–36 months. Next, add in the fact that you may be solely responsible for caring for a newborn baby for the majority of this time.
>
> How would you like your partner (and support network) to support you during this time? Think about how your basic needs will be met, particularly if your partner will have to return to work full-time soon after your procedure. Now consider your wider needs, such as your desire for socialisation, adult company and conversation, etc. Discuss this with your partner.

In these early days, it's important to remember that intimacy doesn't always mean physical closeness. Sometimes emotional intimacy and emotional support – being present, communicating and understanding each other's challenges – are the most vital forms of connection. By nurturing your emotional bond, you're giving your relationship the space it needs to evolve alongside your growing family. This partnership, built on mutual care and understanding, will support you both as you find your rhythm together, strengthening the foundation for both your family and your love.

Breastfeeding demands so much of a mother's time and energy. For the first few months or years, your little one might nurse every few hours. The constant presence of your child can make it difficult to maintain the same kind of one-on-one intimacy you once had with your partner. In a society where partnerships are expected to share duties equally, breastfeeding can often make one parent feel more involved in baby care while the other may feel excluded or left behind.

The expectation that both partners should contribute equally to every aspect of child-rearing can be at odds with breastfeeding, as the mother is often the primary feeder. This can be an emotional strain. There is a deep sense of connection with your baby during feeding moments, and your energy can feel fully consumed by this role – being touched in other ways can feel intrusive, and this is very normal. This change can challenge your connection, and it's important to communicate openly to navigate this. Here are some questions to help open a productive conversation between you and your partner:

Talking Points for Couples

- What are our individual needs during this phase of our relationship?

- How do we both feel about the division of labour in caring for our baby, when it comes to breastfeeding or pumping?

- What adjustments can we make to support each other and avoid resentment?

- How can your partner support you in your breastfeeding or pumping routine?

These conversations can be uncomfortable, but they are key to understanding each other's perspectives and maintaining a solid partnership.

By approaching these challenges with compassion, understanding and a willingness to adapt, you'll be better equipped to navigate the complexities of maintaining intimacy and connection while raising your little one. And remember, this season, with all its ups and downs, is just one chapter in the story of your relationship and your journey as a family.

How Breastfeeding Hormones Affect You and Your Libido

Breastfeeding and Physical Intimacy

Breastfeeding hormones play a significant role in a mother's emotional and physical state. The hormone oxytocin, known as the 'love hormone', is released during breastfeeding and promotes bonding between you and your baby. However, oxytocin also has a calming effect, often leading to feelings of contentment and protectiveness over your baby. This surge in oxytocin can affect how you interact with your partner. You might feel more attuned to your baby's needs and these protective instincts can shift your focus entirely onto your child – your partner may feel they have lost their priority in your eyes.

Breastfeeding can also affect your desire for intimacy. Prolactin, the hormone responsible for milk production can suppress sexual desire during the breastfeeding period. For some mothers, this dip in libido is temporary and returns as breastfeeding or pumping sessions become less frequent. For others, a lower desire for intimacy may persist for as long as they continue nursing.

Beyond hormonal shifts, early motherhood – and breastfeeding in particular – can leave many of us feeling 'touched out' after having a baby quite literally attached to us morning, noon and night. By the time evening rolls around, the idea of more physical closeness might feel overwhelming rather than appealing. It's completely normal if getting busy in the bedroom is the last thing on your mind at the end of a long day of parenting.

It's important to acknowledge these shifts without feeling pressure to 'snap back' into your pre-pregnancy self. Your body, your hormones and your energy are all adjusting and there is no timeline for how long these changes should last. Partners should be sensitive to these shifts, understanding that intimacy may look different during this phase of life.

Talking Points for Couples

- How do you feel about the changes in your intimacy and libido since your baby was born?
- What physical and emotional changes are you experiencing and how can your partner support you through them?
- How can you both find ways to nurture your connection, even if your libido is not where it used to be?

Understanding and accepting these changes is key to maintaining a healthy relationship during the breastfeeding journey.

Maintaining Intimacy in the Face of Change

It's common for couples to feel disconnected during the early days of parenthood, especially when breastfeeding demands take up so much of a mother's time and energy. However, there are many ways to maintain intimacy and connection with your partner, even when you're navigating the complexities of parenthood.

- **Communication is Key:** Open and honest communication is the foundation of a healthy relationship, particularly during times of change. Express how you're feeling without placing blame and be open about what you need from your partner. This could mean discussing physical affection, emotional support or practical help around the house. Share your thoughts on intimacy and any concerns you might have – whether related to breastfeeding, sleep deprivation or any other challenges.

- **Adjust Expectations:** The reality of a romantic relationship changes after the arrival of a baby. The intense physical connection that often exists in the early stages of a relationship may take a backseat as both partners adjust to the new roles of parents. This doesn't mean the relationship is doomed; rather, it's about adapting and finding new ways to nurture the bond. Intimacy doesn't always have to be sexual. It can be found in the moments of quiet connection or holding hands as you walk together.

- **Physical Affection:** Sometimes, the need for closeness is more about physical affection than sex. A cuddle on the couch, gentle touch or even simply being close to your partner can help maintain intimacy. It's important to find what feels good for both of you. As your baby grows and your breastfeeding journey evolves, these moments of physical affection will help strengthen your emotional bond.

Intimacy During Lactation

While it's common to hear about couples navigating shifts in intimacy during breastfeeding, it's important to recognise that every relationship is unique. For some, breastfeeding may bring unexpected challenges to their love life, while for others, it takes nothing away and may even deepen their sense of closeness and connection. Some couples find that breastfeeding enhances intimacy in new ways, while others prefer to keep it separate from their sexual relationship. There is no right or wrong approach – only what feels comfortable and authentic for *you*.

Remember, this is a time of transition and your relationship will evolve as you and your partner continue to find what works for you.

Talking Points for Couples

- How do you both feel about breastfeeding and its impact on your intimacy?

- What boundaries, if any, do you have regarding breastfeeding and sexual activity?

- How can you both respect each other's physical and emotional needs during this time?

The most important takeaway here is that there's no right or wrong way to approach intimacy while breastfeeding. What works for one couple may not work for another, and that's okay. The key is finding a balance that makes both partners feel respected, loved and cared for.

Your Family Dynamics

It's not just your relationship with your romantic partner that changes; your relationship with family members may also undergo a shift. If you've been the daughter who always steps in to handle family matters, that may not be as feasible anymore. Or at least not in the same way while you are nursing or pumping on demand. Similarly, if you've been the granddaughter who takes the lead in checking in on your grandparents or helping with family gatherings, these responsibilities may need to be adjusted during this season of motherhood.

Breastfeeding, and the constant attention it requires, can make it challenging to maintain your usual roles in the family. And that's okay. It's important to give yourself permission to change the way you show up for others. For instance, perhaps you were always the one who organised and hosted family birthday parties before you became a mother – but for now, you simply no longer have the capacity to do so. Communicating your new boundaries and needs with your loved ones is key. By doing so, you allow space for both you and your family to adapt to this new chapter, so that the relationships that matter most to you can continue to thrive in a way that honours your needs as a mother.

Your Friendships

Breastfeeding can also have a significant impact on your friendships, especially as you navigate your parenting choices. If you are breastfeeding beyond the early baby months, in societies where breastfeeding past a few months is not the norm, friends may not fully understand the depth of your commitment or the demands it places on your time and energy. If your friends have preconceived judgments or preconceptions about breastfeeding, it can create tension, especially if they don't share the same values or experiences when it comes to raising children.

Ideally, your friendships are strong enough to weather differences of opinion and parenting choices, but this isn't always the case. Parenting, and especially decisions about how we feed our babies, are incredibly emotive topics. We are all deeply invested in making the best decisions for our families and those choices might look very different from those of even our closest friends. This difference can sometimes create unspoken friction. For example, if you are breastfeeding, your friends who formula-feed might not fully understand why you can't be as spontaneous with social plans or why you can't leave your baby with a sitter for long periods of time.

Friends who don't have children may struggle to grasp just how much time, effort and energy is required to care for and nurture a baby around the clock. They may not realise that the seemingly simple act of going out requires extensive preparation, and even then, leaving your baby can bring about feelings of guilt or anxiety. They may ask why you can't just 'make time for girls' night', without understanding that your baby's needs, especially for breastfeeding, make such outings more complicated.

These differences in understanding can put strain on friendships, but it's essential to communicate openly with your friends about your reality. Acknowledging that your priorities have shifted and that your time is no longer as flexible as it once was, can help create a space for your friends to understand, even if they can't fully relate. Compassionate communication can allow you to maintain your friendships while also prioritising your new role as a mother.

Setting Boundaries with Friends and Family

As we touched upon in Chapter Five (see page 200), one of the biggest challenges of breastfeeding isn't just the physical and emotional demands – it's also managing the well-intentioned (and sometimes unsolicited) opinions of those around you. Whether it's family members questioning how long you plan to breastfeed, friends struggling to understand why your schedule now revolves around feeding or colleagues who don't grasp the logistics of pumping at work, setting clear boundaries can help protect your peace.

If a loved one expresses discomfort or disapproval about your breastfeeding choices, it can be helpful to have a go-to response that acknowledges their feelings but also affirms your decision. Here are some examples of how you might set boundaries in a kind but firm way:

- **To a persistent relative:** 'I appreciate you sharing your thoughts, but I've made an informed decision about breastfeeding, and I'm happy with it. Please don't keep trying to change my mind.'

- **To a friend struggling to understand your availability:** 'I'd love to spend time with you! Right now, my little one's feeding needs make it hard to be as spontaneous as I used to be, but let's find a time that works for both of us.'

- **To a family member questioning night feeds:** 'I know night feeding seems exhausting, but it's actually a natural part of breastfeeding. My baby's sleep patterns will shift in their own time, and I'm comfortable with our current routine.'

Setting these boundaries doesn't mean shutting people out – it means making space for your needs as a breastfeeding mother while still nurturing your relationships in a way that feels right for you.

The Evolving Nature of Relationships While Breastfeeding

Breastfeeding is more than just a way of feeding your baby – it's a deeply transformative experience that can reshape your relationships in unexpected ways. It can bring you closer to your partner or it may require extra effort to maintain intimacy. It can strengthen your bonds with family and friends, but it may also challenge long-standing dynamics. Through open communication, mutual understanding and clear boundaries, you can navigate these changes with grace and confidence.

More than anything, breastfeeding is a season of adaptation – and the same is true for the relationships in your life. While some friendships and family connections will adjust effortlessly, others may require more conversation, patience and compromise. And that's okay. You are evolving in this role as a mother and it's only natural that your relationships will evolve too.

As we move into the next chapter, we'll explore another significant transition: returning to work as a breastfeeding mother. Whether you're planning to continue breastfeeding, pump at work or navigate conversations with your employer, we'll cover practical strategies to help you balance your professional and breastfeeding journey with confidence.

CHAPTER EIGHT

Navigating the Transition Back to Work

Returning to work after having a baby is a significant transition and feels especially complicated when you're breastfeeding. There is a common misconception that you must wean your baby or toddler from breastfeeding before returning to paid employment. This myth is a major reason why the vast majority of UK mothers stop breastfeeding before they are truly ready. I consider myself fortunate to have been able to nurse my son on my own terms for as long as I wanted, but our journey wasn't without its challenges. Returning to work was undoubtedly one of them – just as it has been for many of my clients. But with knowledge comes power and this chapter is all about helping you create a plan to continue breastfeeding, regardless of your working hours. Whether that involves pumping, combination feeding or using supplementary donor milk, this chapter will leave you empowered to make the right choices for you, your family and your unique circumstances.

The decision to return to work at a particular time may not have been your choice, as it wasn't for me. However, pretending to be happy about going back to work when you're actually dreading it is neither healthy nor helpful. Granting yourself permission to be honest about your thoughts, feelings, hopes and fears concerning returning to work while breastfeeding is incredibly important. It may be difficult, but it's incredibly worthwhile.

Denying or suppressing those emotions might seem easier in the short-term, but not acknowledging them can create mental barriers that may make your transition more difficult.

Let's take a moment to be brutally honest about everything you're feeling when it comes to returning to paid employment. Are you excited about doing something that's just for you? Are you terrified about how your baby will nap in your absence? The questions below will help guide you through this process. Use these prompts and make notes in a journal or on your phone or tablet. Then share your answers with someone you love and trust – someone who will listen without judgment and help you reflect on everything you've written.

Journalling Prompts for Returning to Work While Breastfeeding

- **Emotional Readiness**
    - How does thinking about returning to work while breastfeeding make you feel?
    - What emotions come up when you think about balancing work and breastfeeding – excitement, fear, relief, guilt?
    - How do you feel about being away from your little one for longer periods during the day?

- **Practical Considerations**
    - What are your breastfeeding goals once you return to work?
    - Will you pump at work, continue breastfeeding only when home or introduce formula/milk alternatives?

- o What support do you need from your employer to make breastfeeding or pumping feasible?
- o What workplace policies exist for breastfeeding mothers and do you need to request any accommodations?

- **Logistics & Planning**
  - o How will you manage milk expression at work? Will you have time and space to pump?
  - o What is your plan for storing expressed milk?
  - o If your baby doesn't accept a bottle, what alternative feeding methods can you try?
  - o What kind of childcare arrangements feel best for your baby and your family?

- **Work-Life Balance & Boundaries**
  - o How do you want your working hours to fit into your family life?
  - o What (if any) adjustments can you make to ease the transition (e.g. part-time work, hybrid working, flexible start times)?
  - o What are your non-negotiables when it comes to work-life balance?
  - o How will you handle days when you feel torn between work and motherhood?

- **Communication & Support**
  - o What do you need from your employer, partner or support network to make this transition smoother?

- Who can you turn to when you need encouragement and support?
- How can you communicate your needs and boundaries to family, friends and colleagues?

♦ Boundary-setting with Friends & Colleagues

- How will you respond if someone tells you that 'You'll have to stop breastfeeding once you're back at work'?
- If a friend or coworker questions why you're still breastfeeding, how do you want to respond?
- How will you handle situations where you need to pump or take a break for breastfeeding-related needs at work?
- If a colleague or manager seems unsupportive, how can you advocate for your rights while maintaining professionalism?

The law surrounding breastfeeding and returning to work varies widely from place to place, so it's important to be aware of your rights. In the UK, for example, while you have the right to breastfeed in public without discrimination and may request flexible working arrangements or health and safety adjustments, there is no explicit statutory right to breastfeed when you return to work. However, many employers have breastfeeding policies, so it's worth finding out whether your workplace has one. For more information, visit www.acas.org.uk.

Speak to your employer about your intention to continue breastfeeding once you return to work. This is important even if you work from home or don't anticipate breastfeeding affecting your work day. There may come a time when you need to express milk, pump or nurse your baby during working hours.

Questions to Ask Your Employer About Pumping at Work

Advocating for your needs as a breastfeeding mother in the workplace can feel daunting, but open communication with your employer can help set clear expectations and ensure a smooth transition. Here are some key questions to guide your discussion:

Workplace Policies & Legal Rights

- Does our workplace have a formal breastfeeding or pumping policy?
- What accommodations does the company offer for breastfeeding employees?
- Has a risk assessment been conducted to ensure a safe and supportive environment for nursing or pumping mothers?

Pumping Location & Privacy

- Is there a private, clean space (other than a bathroom) where I can pump during the work day? (Or) Will I have access to a lockable or designated lactation room?
- If no dedicated space exists, is there a way to arrange a temporary private space for pumping?

Time & Scheduling for Pumping

- Can I take short breaks to pump during the work day? If so, how often and for how long?
- Can I adjust my work schedule to accommodate pumping sessions (e.g. flexible start times, remote work options or compressed hours)?

- If I need to pump at specific times, how can we integrate this into my workload without disrupting my productivity?

Milk Storage & Logistics

- Is there a refrigerator available for breast milk storage or should I bring my own cooler?
- Can I bring and store my breast pump on-site safely?

Workload & Performance Expectations

- How will my pumping schedule be accommodated in relation to meetings and deadlines?
- Can I have input into my workload distribution to ensure my responsibilities remain manageable?

Colleague Awareness & Inclusivity

- Will my need to pump be communicated to relevant colleagues to avoid unnecessary interruptions or scheduling conflicts?
- How does our workplace support a culture of inclusivity for breastfeeding mothers?

Additional Support & Resources

- Are there any employee resource groups, HR representatives or workplace wellness programmes that support breastfeeding employees?
- Would the company consider implementing or updating a formal breastfeeding-friendly policy if one does not exist?

These questions can serve as a starting point for an open, productive discussion with your employer. The goal is not to seek permission to breastfeed but to create a supportive work environment that enables you to continue your breastfeeding journey while fulfilling your professional responsibilities.

How to Breastfeed as a Working Mum

Preparing Your Baby for the Transition

If you plan to continue breastfeeding after returning to work, introducing a bottle or alternative feeding method ahead of time can make the transition smoother for both you and your baby. While some babies adapt easily, others may initially resist taking milk from a bottle, particularly if they have been exclusively breastfed.

One technique that can help is paced bottle feeding, which more closely mimics the natural rhythm of breastfeeding. This method encourages your baby to take the bottle in a way that supports oral development and prevents overfeeding. If your baby is new to bottle feeding or if you're concerned about bottle refusal, it may help to introduce this technique before your return to work.

Key principles of paced bottle feeding:

- Use a **slow-flow teat** to keep the milk flow similar to breastfeeding.

- Hold the bottle **horizontally**, allowing your baby to control the flow of milk.

- Let your baby **latch onto the bottle teat** rather than pushing it into their mouth.

- **Pause regularly** during feeds, giving your baby time to swallow, breathe and regulate their intake – just as they would at the breast.

This feeding style is particularly helpful for caregivers who will be feeding your baby in your absence. If possible, allow someone else to give the first few bottles while you're out of sight, as babies often associate breastfeeding with their mother and may refuse a bottle if they sense that nursing is an option.

By introducing paced bottle feeding well in advance, you're giving your baby time to adjust while also helping to protect your breastfeeding relationship by ensuring that bottle feeding does not create a preference for fast milk flow.

Option One (For Babies Under Six Months & Exclusively Breastfed)

If your baby is under six months old and you want to continue exclusively breastfeeding when you return to work, you will most likely need to express milk or pump while you're at work. Exceptions to this would include working fewer than three hours at a time or if you can nurse your baby during breaks, either by travelling to them or having them come to you at work. This could be an option if you're working from home or if your baby is with a caregiver at or near your workplace.

If you plan on travelling to and from your baby during breaks, consider how this will impact your physical and mental health. Is it feasible to take time for travelling, eating, drinking and nursing your baby? Is it possible for the caregiver to bring your baby to you during your break? Be honest with yourself about the practicality of this option.

If you do not nurse your baby on your breaks but still wish to exclusively breastfeed, you will need to express milk for them while at work. You do not need to build an enormous freezer stash before returning to work, but you will need to pump regularly throughout the day to maintain your milk supply and ensure your baby has enough milk.

Research tells us that exclusively breastfed babies consume an average of 750ml (25oz) per day between one and six months old. A typical range is 570–900ml (19–30oz). The variation depends on each baby's individual needs and feeding patterns, but it's important to note that this is for expressed milk, which can differ slightly from what a baby consumes directly from the breast. To calculate the amount of expressed milk your baby will need while you are at work, follow these steps:

1. Estimate how many times your baby breastfeeds per day.
2. Divide 750ml (25oz) by the number of feedings.

This gives you a rough guide for how much expressed milk your baby will need per feeding. For example, if your baby breastfeeds eight times per day, you can estimate they will need around 94ml (3oz) of expressed milk per feeding.

Keep in mind that your baby may nurse more frequently once you're reunited after work. This is normal and will settle as your baby adjusts to your new routine.

Option Two (For Babies Under Six Months & Combi-fed)

If your baby is under six months old and you don't want to pump or express milk while at work, you can introduce formula or donor milk to supplement their diet. If you're considering donor milk, check your local milk bank for availability.

How to Introduce Formula

When introducing formula, follow the manufacturer's instructions for preparation and gradually increase the amount that you add to your baby's bottle. Start with 75% breast milk and 25% formula, then gradually replace more breast milk with formula over time. It typically takes 3–5 days for your breasts to adjust to each feed you drop, but your baby may take longer to adapt to the change.

Be sure to practise paced, responsive bottle feeding to prevent overfeeding and ask your child's caregiver to do the same. You will notice a drop in your milk supply once you introduce formula, which is completely normal. Your supply should adjust to your new routine within 5–7 days. Until it does, you may need to express small amounts of milk for your comfort only – even if you don't plan on expressing milk regularly at work. To do this, only express as much milk as you need to in order to feel comfortable, rather than emptying your breasts completely (which will stimulate your milk production). Head to Chapter Three for more information on managing your milk supply (see page 74).

Option Three (For Babies Over Six Months & Breastfed Alongside Solids, No Pumping)

If your baby is over six months old and you want to continue breastfeeding without pumping or introducing formula, you can breastfeed before and after work while your baby consumes solids and water during the day. However, this will only work if you're away from your baby for a limited amount of time and if your baby is eating solids well.

If you are away from your baby overnight or for extended hours, they will need additional milk – whether expressed, donor milk or formula – during your absence.

Option Four (For Babies Over Six Months & Breastfed and Pumped Alongside Solids)

If your baby is over six months old and you're planning to express milk for them while you're at work, you'll need to have a freezer stash of milk or pump regularly while away. For day one, aim to leave a maximum of six 90ml (3oz) bottles of expressed milk, adjusting based on how much your baby consumes.

Trust that even if your baby doesn't consume much expressed milk while you're away, they will have solid foods and water. When you reunite, they may nurse longer to make up for the missed feedings – this is completely normal and will help maintain your supply.

How to Deal with Bottle Refusal

A common concern for breastfeeding mothers returning to work is that their baby may refuse to take a bottle of expressed milk or formula in their absence. While some babies transition seamlessly, others strongly prefer nursing at the breast and may initially resist bottle feeding.

If this happens, don't panic – your baby will not starve themselves. They may simply need time to adjust. Here are some practical steps you can take:

- **Ensure caregivers are using paced bottle feeding.** Discussed earlier in this chapter (see page 233), this method helps your baby adjust more easily by slowing the milk flow and mirroring breastfeeding rhythms.

- **Have someone else offer the bottle.** Babies often refuse bottles if they know breastfeeding is an option.

- **Experiment with different bottle types or alternative feeding methods.** Try feeding with a sippy cup, open cup, syringe or spoon – especially for babies over six months.

- **Offer milk when your baby is calm rather than very hungry.** Frustration can make them more resistant to a new feeding method.

- **Try different holding positions.** Some babies prefer to be bottle-fed in a different position from breastfeeding to avoid confusion.

For most babies bottle refusal is temporary. If your little one still struggles, a local breastfeeding counsellor or lactation consultant can offer personalised advice based on your baby's age and feeding patterns.

Timing is also essential when introducing a bottle. While it might feel urgent, try not to rush the process. When you first try to introduce a bottle to your baby it can be stressful. I first tried when my baby was five months and I worried that he'd be starving! Thankfully, he drank a small amount in my absence and eagerly nursed when I returned. If this happens to you, don't worry. It's normal for the first attempts to be challenging, particularly if it's you offering a bottle and expecting them to accept when they are used to breastfeeding from you. Early attempts may be better made by the non-breastfeeding partner. The key is to stay calm and patient, remembering that your baby's preferences may take time to adjust.

Start Slow and Be Patient

The first few bottle-feeding attempts may not go as planned and that's okay. Babies are creatures of habit and it may take a little while for them to adapt to something new. Start by offering a small amount of milk when your baby is calm, but not too hungry. This lowers the stress level and increases the chances of them accepting the bottle. Try to create a calm, nurturing environment during the process. If your baby refuses, don't push it – take a break and try again later.

Choosing the Right Bottle and Teat

Selecting the right bottle and teat can make all the difference. While a slow-flow teat is often recommended for most babies, it's important to experiment with different types of nipples and bottles to find the best fit for your baby. Some babies may prefer teats that are more slow-flowing, while others may do better with a faster-flowing teat. If your baby struggles with the standard teats, try different options until you find one that works. Keep in mind that every baby is different and some trial and error is normal.

Alternatives to Bottles

If you're concerned about nipple confusion or want to explore alternatives, consider options like sippy cups, open cups or even using a spoon or syringe for feeding smaller amounts. While bottles are convenient, they're not always the best long-term solution, especially as your baby's teeth and jaw develop. When your baby is around one, you can gradually introduce sippy cups or open cups to promote oral health and give them a new way of drinking.

Make it a Positive Experience

It's essential to keep the experience as positive as possible. Babies are very in tune with their caregivers' emotions, so try to remain calm and reassuring during the process. Speak softly to your baby and hold them close to create a secure environment. If you're still facing difficulties, it might help to have someone else offer the bottle, as babies may associate you with breastfeeding and resist bottle feeding when you're the one offering it.

Remember, patience is key. Even if your baby refuses the bottle at first it doesn't mean they won't come around. Stick with it and try not to stress. Eventually, with consistency and support your baby will adjust. You are giving them a positive foundation for future feeding, and with each attempt, you're helping them adapt to the new routine.

What is a Freezer Stash?

A freezer stash is simply any breast milk that you have stored in your freezer for future use. Many mothers feel that they need a huge freezer stash to continue breastfeeding their baby or toddler once they return to work, but this is not necessarily the case. If you are exclusively pumping, you may plan to build up a larger stash before you go back to work. Alternatively, you may want to create a stash if you won't be able to pump regularly at work but would like your baby or toddler to have expressed milk while they are with other caregivers.

As with every aspect of breastfeeding, it's important to remember that everyone's journey is unique and what works for one person may not work for another. When considering whether to build a freezer stash, ask yourself the following questions to help guide your decision:

- Will you realistically be able to pump regularly before returning to work?

- Do you have a safe and effective way to store breast milk?

- Is pumping likely to have a negative impact on your physical or mental health?

> **Tips for Building a Freezer Stash**
>
> 1. **Consider parallel pumping.** This means pumping from the opposite breast to the one that you are nursing your baby from, as you feed. You can use any type of pump to do this.
>
> 2. **Consider wearing milk shells** in between feeds to catch any milk that would ordinarily be absorbed by breast milk pads.
>
> 3. **Pump after feeding your baby.** This will increase your milk supply while you are still feeding your baby at the breast. This allows your baby to satisfy their hunger and thirst at the breast first so that you are primarily feeding your baby and not the freezer.
>
> 4. **Follow my tips for maximum pumping effectiveness** in Chapter Two (see page 109).
>
> 5. **Give yourself permission for your best to be more than enough.** Remember that your baby needs a happy and healthy mother more than they need your breast milk.

Reverse Cycling: Why It Happens and How to Navigate It

Reverse cycling can be one of the most challenging aspects of returning to work as a nursing mother. It's a term that refers to some babies' natural adjustment to feeding less during the day when their mother is away and then compensating by nursing more frequently at night.

Why Does Reverse Cycling Happen?

Reverse cycling often occurs when a baby:

- Prefers to wait for the breast rather than taking a bottle while separated from their mother.
- Feeds less during the day due to distractions, a change in routine or separation.
- Seeks extra comfort and connection through night nursing, especially during transitions like returning to work.
- Is going through a developmental leap or a growth spurt, which increases their need for milk and closeness.

While reverse cycling can be exhausting, it's usually temporary. It's your baby's way of adapting to this new routine while still maintaining their breastfeeding relationship. If you find yourself navigating this pattern, here are some tried-and-tested tips that can help:

1. **Maximise Time with Your Child:** When you're home, focus exclusively on your baby as much as possible. Create as many opportunities as you can for one-on-one connection during waking hours to help reduce the need for that connection-seeking overnight. Simple activities like reading books together, baby massage, giving 100 kisses, tickle time or other bonding moments can be effective ways to reconnect after a day apart.

2. **Family Bedtime:** Consider going to sleep at the same time as your baby (and/or older children) to maximise your sleep, especially during the first half of the night. This may mean sacrificing watching the latest series

on Netflix or having evening time with your partner. If possible, aim to get as much sleep as you can before midnight – this can be incredibly impactful until reverse cycling settles down.

3. **Share the Night Shift:** If you have a partner or family who can help, ask them to take at least part of the night shift, especially if your baby is more wakeful than sleepy. This may allow you to get at least four hours of uninterrupted sleep.

You at Work

Actively give yourself permission to be fully present once you return to work, rather than constantly checking your phone for updates from your childcare provider every ten minutes. This is, of course, easier said than done, but it will make your work day feel smoother and go by more quickly. Focussing on your work will not only help you be more productive, but it will also stop the day feeling like it's dragging on. Remember to give yourself permission to not feel guilty about being away from your little one during working hours. Assuming you don't have pre-existing supply issues, your milk supply will adjust, allowing you to continue breastfeeding around your work schedule, if that is your choice.

Give yourself time and space to adjust. You may find that you enjoy being back at work more than you expected, or perhaps your feelings about your job have changed now that you are a mother. Whatever emotions arise, give yourself permission to express them openly and honestly with someone you trust, whether that's in person, online or via voice notes. Feelings of guilt and inner conflict are common, but it may help to remind yourself why you're returning to work and to consider the alternative for both you and your family if you didn't.

If returning to work simply feels like too much, take a step back and explore your options with your partner and support network, if you have one. Can you make sacrifices to spend more time at home? It may be worth considering whether a temporary shift in your work situation or family dynamics could make this possible. However, if returning to your job is non-negotiable, work on recognising that you are truly doing the best for your family every single day. Acknowledge the sacrifices you are making and take pride in them.

Find your at-work-mama-crew with whom you can share the highs and lows of being a working mum. This may mean a slight shift in your former working relationships, and that's okay. It is not a crime to develop new friendships as you evolve into your mother edition.

Drink your baby in with reckless abandon upon your reunions. Even if it is only for 15 minutes before their bedtime, give yourself and them the gift of one-to-one focussed time when you kiss, cuddle and nurse your bundle of love. The rush of oxytocin that you both feel will put even the toughest day at work into perspective. Once more, allow yourself to be fully present and with them for an undisturbed period, if possible. The quality of the time that you spend together matters so very much.

How to Manage a Trip Away from Your Breastfed Baby or Toddler

If you're preparing for a work trip, you might feel torn between the excitement of a little time away and the anxiety about leaving your nursling overnight. You may find yourself going back and forth between the thought of some well-deserved me-time and the concern about how your little one will cope without you. These feelings are completely normal, and it's okay to feel both ways at different times. The reality of managing a trip away from your baby is full of practical questions you'll need to address to make your time apart as smooth as possible for both of you. Let's dive into those burning questions, from managing your milk supply to ensuring your baby is comforted and nourished.

How to Manage Your Milk Supply & Avoid Engorgement

If your baby is under three months old, your milk supply is still heavily influenced by your hormones. A short trip away, even a couple of days, may not cause lasting changes, but you will likely need to pump or express milk to avoid engorgement and prevent clogged ducts. If your baby is older than three months, your milk supply will be more influenced by the frequency with which you remove milk. Being away for more than two or three days could cause a slight, temporary dip in supply, so try to pump or express milk at intervals that mirror your baby's usual nursing times. If you have access to a freezer and cooler bag you can store milk for your baby's future use, keeping their feeding routine as consistent as possible.

How Will My Baby Be Comforted & Fall Asleep Without Being Nursed?

If your baby usually falls asleep while breastfeeding, you might be worried about how they'll manage in your absence. But here's the good news: babies can fall asleep without nursing if they feel safe and comfortable. For a successful transition, ensure that your baby's caregiver understands and follows the soothing bedtime routine you've established. If your baby is used to being nursed to sleep, practise comforting methods with your caregiver beforehand, such as rocking, patting or singing to help your baby settle. The key is to provide a consistent, familiar environment.

Creating a comforting sleep space that mirrors the usual routine is helpful. For example, some babies benefit from a darkened room, a consistent bedtime story or gentle rocking. If your partner or caregiver is less familiar with the bedtime routine, ensure they have plenty of opportunities to practise soothing your baby, even if it's just with naps. The more comfortable your caregiver is, the easier the transition will be.

Should I Wean My Child Off the Breast Before Going Away?

A common myth is that you should wean your child before leaving on a trip, but this is generally unnecessary and can create more stress for both you and your baby. Ideally, weaning should be a gradual, gentle process. Whatever your return to paid employment looks like, recognise that everything you do is for your child(ren). Every action, every decision you make is made with their well-being in mind. You are quite literally doing the most, every day, 24/7. So, take a moment to give yourself the credit you truly deserve. Finally, give yourself permission to wean once you return to work or at any point if you feel it is the right choice for you and your family. Head to Chapter Ten (see page 265) for support to do this gently and responsively and not in a way that's rushed for the sake of a trip.

Abrupt weaning can result in discomfort, engorgement and hormonal shifts, not to mention confusion for your baby. If breastfeeding is an important source of comfort for both of you, taking a break from nursing during a trip doesn't need to be the end of that connection. When you return, breastfeeding can resume to reconnect and reassure your baby that your bond remains strong.

Preparing for Your Time Away

Preparing your child and their caregiver ahead of your trip can make all the difference in how smoothly things go. If your baby or toddler is used to being comforted by you, provide your caregiver with all the information they need about your child's preferences for sleep, feeding and soothing. If your partner or caregiver hasn't spent much time alone with your baby, consider doing a 'rehearsal' nap or overnight stay in advance. This will give both your child and their caregiver the opportunity to adjust and feel more confident.

Prep Checklist

- Review your child's feeding schedule and ensure there's enough milk/formula for their needs.
- Establish a comforting sleep routine and share it with the caregiver.
- Give your child and caregiver time to practise comforting methods.
- Pack any necessary feeding, sleep and comfort items.
- Make a plan for maintaining milk supply, including expressing or pumping while you're away.

With a little preparation and confidence in your child's adaptability, your time away can be an enriching experience for both you and your baby. When you're reunited, that first feed will feel even more rewarding, knowing you've both navigated this temporary separation with care and love.

Closing Thoughts

Returning to work while breastfeeding is undeniably a journey of balancing many emotions and responsibilities. It's a dance of finding ways to nourish not only your baby but also yourself, all while fulfilling your professional obligations. But remember, this doesn't mean you have to sacrifice your bond with your baby or your well-being. There are no perfect formulas for this balance – what matters most is that you listen to *your* body, trust *your* instincts and embrace the choices that work best for *your* unique family.

You are not alone in this; there's an entire community of mothers who understand, and who are walking similar paths. So, take a deep breath, trust yourself and remember: you are not just managing work and breastfeeding – you are showing your child the power of resilience, balance and love. That is more than enough, and so are you.

CHAPTER NINE

Breastfeeding, Menstruation, Fertility and Pregnancy

Breastfeeding can have a profound impact on your menstrual cycle, fertility and even future pregnancies. However, misinformation surrounding these topics can lead to confusion, unnecessary worry and even premature weaning.

In this chapter, we will dispel common myths and provide evidence-based information on:

- How breastfeeding affects the return of menstruation and what to expect.

- The relationship between breastfeeding and fertility, including natural birth spacing.

- Breastfeeding during pregnancy – what's safe, what might change and how to manage it.

- Tandem breastfeeding – nursing an older child while feeding a newborn.

By understanding how breastfeeding interacts with your reproductive cycle, you can make informed choices that support both your feeding journey and your long-term family-planning goals.

Breastfeeding and Your Period

During breastfeeding your body produces high levels of prolactin – the hormone responsible for milk production – which can suppress ovulation and menstruation. Prolactin can also prevent the lining of your uterus from thickening enough to support a new pregnancy. This natural process is called lactational amenorrhoea and is part of nature's way of spacing out births. As a result, some mothers may not experience a period for months or even years, for as long as they are breastfeeding. For others, the return of menstruation may occur earlier, particularly if they are not exclusively breastfeeding or their baby begins to consume more solid foods.

It's important to remember that the return of your period does not signal a permanent decrease in milk supply, nor does it mean that your breastfeeding relationship is coming to an end. However, some mothers may notice a temporary dip in their milk production when their period returns. This is because the fluctuating hormones that accompany ovulation and menstruation can affect your prolactin levels. If this happens, don't panic – it's usually short-lived, and there are steps you can take to support your milk supply during this time.

The timing of your period's return depends on several factors, including the frequency and intensity of your breastfeeding. If you're breastfeeding on demand, particularly at night, your prolactin levels will remain elevated, which may keep your period at bay for longer. Conversely, as your baby begins to sleep for longer stretches or consume more solids, your prolactin levels may decrease, which can trigger the return of ovulation and your period.

Managing the Return of Your Period

When your period does return, it may not be as predictable or regular at first. If you do notice a decrease in your milk supply around the time of your period, stay hydrated and try to eat enough nutrient-dense foods to ensure that you're getting enough nutrients to support your milk production. Magnesium and calcium are particularly important. Magnesium plays a role in your prolactin production and calcium is essential for your milk production too. Ensuring that you are getting enough of these minerals can help minimise supply fluctuations. Magnesium-rich foods like leafy greens, nuts, seeds and calcium-rich foods like dairy products, fortified plant milks and tofu can all help too.

Breastfeeding and Your Fertility

It's important to recognise that ovulation occurs before menstruation, so even if your period has not returned and you are breastfeeding, you could still be fertile. With this in mind, if you're not ready to conceive again, be sure to use contraception to avoid an unintended pregnancy. Yes, breastfeeding can provide natural contraception, but it's not foolproof, especially if your baby is eating solid foods or breastfeeding less frequently. If you're not ready to conceive again, you should definitely use another form of contraception alongside breastfeeding. Speak to your family doctor about your options as a nursing or pumping mum.

Journeying Through Pregnancy While Breastfeeding

Whether you dreamed of nursing through pregnancy or it comes as one of motherhood's many surprises, the decision to breastfeed during pregnancy can be both beautiful and challenging, offering a unique opportunity to nourish both your growing baby and your toddler or older child at the same time. However, it also brings its own set of physical, emotional and logistical considerations. It's important to approach this experience with compassion for yourself, a nurturing mindset and realistic expectations. Understanding the challenges and joys of breastfeeding during pregnancy will help you make informed decisions that are best for you and your family.

Embarking on the journey of pregnancy while continuing to breastfeed your young child is a deeply personal decision that requires careful consideration. Some research suggests that breastfeeding during pregnancy *may* be associated with an increased risk of miscarriage, particularly when breastfeeding is exclusive – meaning the baby relies solely on breast milk for nutrition. However, studies show that no increased risk has been observed with complementary breastfeeding – that is, when your child also consumes solid foods or other milk sources alongside breastfeeding. In fact, many mothers continue to breastfeed successfully throughout their pregnancy, adjusting as needed to changes in their milk production and their child's feeding patterns.

When you become pregnant while still breastfeeding, your body faces the awesome task of supporting both your growing baby and your nursing child. As a pregnant mother, you need more nutrients than non-pregnant women, as you are not only supporting the developing baby in your womb but also producing breast milk. As your pregnancy progresses, your energy needs rise and it can sometimes feel like an overwhelming balancing act. However, your body *is* capable of incredible things, and with the right nourishment, rest and support, many mothers continue to breastfeed through pregnancy while staying strong and well.

Breastfeeding Through Pregnancy: Challenges, Changes and Choices

Breastfeeding while pregnant is a unique experience that can bring both joy and challenges. Some mothers continue nursing throughout pregnancy without difficulty, while others experience physical discomfort, emotional shifts or a desire to set new boundaries. Understanding what to expect can help you navigate this journey with confidence and self-compassion.

Physical and Emotional Considerations

As your pregnancy progresses, hormonal fluctuations – especially rising oestrogen and progesterone levels – can lead to sore breasts, nipple sensitivity or nursing aversion. Some mothers find that breastfeeding becomes uncomfortable or even unbearable, while others feel no significant changes. Additionally, nursing mothers' milk supply often decreases in the second trimester, which may naturally lead to weaning or a reduced interest in breastfeeding from their older child.

Beyond the physical aspects, breastfeeding while pregnant can bring up a range of emotions. Some mothers feel a deep sense of connection and comfort through nursing, while others experience sheer frustration or exhaustion. Both experiences are completely normal, and it's essential to acknowledge and accept your feelings and needs throughout the process.

Setting Boundaries and Weaning Considerations

If breastfeeding begins to feel overwhelming while you are pregnant, setting nursing boundaries can help you maintain a balance that works for both you and your child. This might mean:

- Reducing the number of feeds or gradually shortening nursing sessions.
- Limiting feeding to certain times of day, such as before naps or bedtime.
- Encouraging other sources of comfort, such as cuddling, reading or gentle rocking.

Some mothers decide to wean completely during pregnancy, while others continue nursing until their child naturally loses interest. There is no right or wrong choice – only what feels best for you and your family. If you do choose to stop, weaning gradually can make the transition smoother for both you and your child. If you would like to introduce breastfeeding boundaries, or stop breastfeeding during pregnancy, head to Chapter Ten for more information (see page 265).

The Beauty of Breastfeeding Through Pregnancy

While some women find breastfeeding through pregnancy challenging, others experience it as a deeply nurturing and positive journey. For some, nursing remains a powerful source of comfort and connection, helping both mother and child adjust to the changes that pregnancy brings.

Ultimately, breastfeeding through pregnancy is a personal decision. Trust your instincts, listen to your body and allow yourself the flexibility to make changes as needed. Whether you continue nursing, set new boundaries or stop breastfeeding, your choice is valid – and what matters most is that you feel supported and at peace with your decision.

Maintaining Your Milk Supply During Pregnancy

As a breastfeeding mother navigating pregnancy, you may have questions and concerns about whether you will continue to produce enough milk for your nursling. The good news is that, for many women, breastfeeding during pregnancy does not drastically impact their milk production. However, it's important to note that as early as 12–16 weeks, pregnancy hormones signal your body to prepare for colostrum production for your growing baby which will change the composition of your milk.

For some toddlers, the taste of colostrum can be unappealing and they may self-wean, while others will continue to nurse as usual. Some mothers find that their milk supply decreases or dries up entirely, while others can continue nursing right up until birth.

Here are some essential nutrients to prioritise:

- **Iron:** Your body needs extra iron to support both your pregnancy and your breastfeeding child. Foods rich in iron include lean meats, leafy greens, lentils, beans, tofu and fortified cereals. Pairing these with vitamin C-rich foods like oranges, tomatoes and bell peppers will help improve iron absorption.

- **Calcium:** To maintain your bone health and support your baby's bone development, make sure to consume plenty of calcium-rich foods like dairy products, fortified plant milks, leafy greens and calcium-fortified tofu.

- **Magnesium:** This mineral supports muscle function and relaxation, helping to manage the physical demands of breastfeeding and pregnancy. Include magnesium-rich foods like nuts, seeds, wholegrains, legumes and dark leafy greens.

- **Vitamins:** During this period, your body requires higher amounts of key vitamins to support both your baby and your milk production. Foods rich in these vitamins include:

    o **Vitamin D:** Found in fatty fish, fortified dairy and sunlight exposure.

    o **Vitamin A:** Found in sweet potatoes, carrots and dark leafy greens.

- **Vitamin C:** Found in citrus fruits, bell peppers, strawberries and tomatoes.

- **B Vitamins:** Found in wholegrains, eggs and lean meats.

While aiming for a balanced and varied diet, let's be real – between parenting, work and all the other demands of life, it can feel impossible to always have three perfectly nutritious meals every day. And that's okay! Life is busy and some days it's not going to be perfect. If you're finding it difficult to meet your nutritional needs with food, you're not alone – and it's absolutely okay to talk to a nutritionist or healthcare professional about prenatal vitamins or supplements that could support you.

Preparing for Birth While Breastfeeding

As you navigate breastfeeding while pregnant, it's important to begin preparing for the arrival of your new baby. This may involve making adjustments to your breastfeeding routine, setting gentle boundaries around nursing or introducing new foods to your older child as your milk supply changes. Preparing your older child for the transition is equally important, as it helps them understand the changes that are coming. Even if your older child is non-verbal, you can help them understand by using books, toys and role-play.

In addition to preparing your child, it's crucial to prepare for the birth itself and ensure you have the right support in place for the postpartum period. Many mothers find that breastfeeding during labour can provide relaxation and comfort, but it's also essential to prioritise your own rest and recovery.

One universal truth is that having a solid support system in place postnatally – whether it's your partner, family, friends or paid support – is absolutely essential. Surrounding yourself with compassionate, reliable help will make the transition to life with a new baby that much smoother, both emotionally and physically.

Compassionate Decision-making

Breastfeeding during pregnancy is a unique journey for each mother. What works for one family may not be the best choice for another. You may find breastfeeding during pregnancy to be an enriching and fulfilling experience, or you may decide that it's simply not the right choice for you. Trust yourself and listen to your body; what matters most is that you make the decisions that are right for you, your family and your well-being.

Be kind to yourself as you make these decisions, too. Whether you choose to continue breastfeeding, introduce boundaries or wean, know that you're doing what's best for your family. There is no one 'right' way to navigate this rollercoaster that we call motherhood and you are doing an incredible job, no matter what. You are not alone, either – I hope you take comfort in the knowledge that many mothers before you have walked this path although *this* journey is uniquely yours.

Tandem Breastfeeding

Nursing your older child and your newborn (or twins, or multiples) can be a beautiful choice for many mothers, though it requires careful consideration of both the physical and emotional aspects for you and your children. The arrival of a new sibling often brings mixed emotions for your older child. They may feel excitement and joy, but they may also experience confusion, jealousy or sadness as their routine shifts, including changes to breastfeeding. This is all normal and it is vital to make space for any negative reactions that your child may have as well as any positive ones.

Tandem nursing can help ease this transition, providing your older child with the comfort, connection and security they need during this big change. However, it can also be physically demanding on your body, especially in the early days of postpartum recovery. Despite this, many mothers find that tandem nursing offers a wonderful opportunity to bond with both children, creating intimate, nurturing moments for everyone. Breast milk remains nutritionally appropriate for both your newborn and older child, with the composition of your milk adapting over time to meet the nutritional needs of both. Aren't you a wonder?

While tandem breastfeeding has many benefits, it can also come with challenges. Some mothers may experience sore nipples, emotional overwhelm or a drop in milk supply as their body adjusts to nursing two children. Let's unpack the realities of tandem nursing over the next few pages.

Deciding Whether to Tandem Feed

For many mums, the decision to tandem feed – breastfeeding an older child alongside a newborn – is not taken lightly. It requires careful thought about personal goals, the needs of both children and how your body feels during and after pregnancy. Some mothers plan to tandem feed from the start, while others find themselves making the decision unexpectedly when their older child shows continued interest in breastfeeding after their new baby arrives.

Additionally, some mothers breastfeed twins or multiples, navigating the unique demands of feeding more than one baby of the same age. Others may nurse children of different ages, balancing the needs of a newborn with those of older children who still seek comfort at the breast.

Why Some Mothers Choose to Tandem Feed

Tandem feeding can be a deeply rewarding experience and may offer several benefits, including:

- Maintaining a strong bond with an older child during the transition of welcoming a new sibling.

- Easing jealousy or sibling rivalry by allowing an older child to continue nursing.

- Providing additional nutrition and comfort for toddlers or preschoolers who still rely on breastfeeding for security.

- Supporting milk supply, as the increased demand from both children can help with milk production in the early postpartum period.

- Helping to manage oversupply or engorgement in the early weeks of postpartum recovery.

Why Some Mothers Choose Not to Tandem Feed

While some mothers find tandem feeding beneficial, others decide against it for personal or practical reasons, such as:

- Physical discomfort, especially if breastfeeding during pregnancy was already challenging.

- Nursing aversion, which can be heightened when feeding two children at once.

- Wanting a clear transition between breastfeeding one child and caring for a newborn.

- Needing a break between breastfeeding journeys, as pregnancy and breastfeeding are so physically demanding – some mothers prefer to give their bodies time to recover.

- ♦ Logistical challenges, such as balancing the needs of multiple children while ensuring the newborn's nutritional needs remain the priority.

Making the Right Choice for You

Every breastfeeding journey is unique, and there is no one-size-fits-all approach. Each mum must decide what aligns with her well-being and her children's needs when it comes to tandem feeding. If you are considering tandem feeding, think about how it aligns with your physical and emotional well-being as well as your children's needs. Setting boundaries, such as limiting nursing sessions for the older child, might help create a balance that works for everyone.

Ultimately, the most important factor in this decision is that you feel supported and confident in your choice, whether you choose to continue breastfeeding multiple children or wean your older child before your new baby arrives. I want to remind you that your body, your comfort and your needs matter, too.

Tandem Feeding: Different Experiences and Considerations

The decision to tandem feed – or to wean an older child during pregnancy – can look different for every mother. Some find the experience rewarding, while others struggle with physical discomfort, changing emotions or shifting dynamics between siblings.

For some mothers, nursing aversion – which we deep dive into in Chapter Four (see page 140) – can be a challenge. One client I worked with, Tish, continued breastfeeding her

12-month-old throughout pregnancy, even as she experienced unexpected feelings of resentment while feeding. After researching, she realised this was a common response to breastfeeding while pregnant, which reassured her. Though it was difficult at times, she remained committed to natural weaning. When her second baby was born, she initially found tandem feeding tricky to manage, often feeding her newborn first before her toddler. Now, with one child 16 months old and the other 37 months, she continues to breastfeed both, though her older child nurses only occasionally as part of a gradual weaning process.

Other mothers experience a natural stopping point before the new baby arrives. Tahni, who I also worked with, noticed that her milk supply had dropped in the third trimester and asked her toddler if they were still getting milk. One night, her toddler simply decided not to nurse, marking the end of their breastfeeding journey. Although she had been struggling with aversion in the final minutes of feeding, letting go was still emotionally difficult for her. After her second baby was born, her toddler occasionally asked to nurse again, but she gently redirected them to other sources of comfort.

These stories highlight the many factors that shape the decision to tandem feed or wean, including:

- **Physical comfort** – Some mothers experience nipple sensitivity, aversion or a drop in milk supply, which can influence their decision.

- **Emotional well-being** – Feelings of resentment, exhaustion or deep attachment to the breastfeeding bond can all impact whether a mother continues or stops.

- **Child-led vs. mother-led weaning** – Some toddlers naturally lose interest, while others continue to seek comfort at the breast. Parents may choose to follow their child's lead or set boundaries based on their own needs.

- **Logistical challenges** – Managing feeds for two children at different stages can be complex, with some mothers prioritising the newborn's needs while maintaining a gradual weaning process for the older child.

Ultimately, there is no single way to breastfeed during pregnancy or tandem feeding – only what feels manageable and sustainable for each mother and her family. Recognising your own needs, setting boundaries where necessary and allowing room for flexibility can make the journey smoother, whatever path you choose.

Journal Prompts to Help You Decide

- What are my personal goals for breastfeeding during this new season of motherhood?
- How do I feel about continuing to breastfeed my older child while also nursing a newborn?
- What are my older child's needs and how does breastfeeding currently support them?
- What physical and emotional challenges am I prepared to navigate, and what support systems do I have in place?

How to Tandem Nurse

Let's explore the various ways that you might tandem breastfeed in ways that work for you and your family.

Approaches to Tandem Nursing

- **One breast for each child:** Assigning each child their own breast can be a helpful strategy for balancing your milk supply and making feeding sessions more predictable. Since each breast responds to the demand placed upon it independently, feeding one child consistently from the same side allows that breast to adjust its supply to their needs.

This means that milk supply can differ between breasts, depending on how often and how effectively each child nurses. For example, if a newborn feeds more frequently than an older sibling, the breast they use may produce a greater volume of milk, with a higher carbohydrate content suited to their growth needs. Meanwhile, the other breast, used by the older child, may produce less but still provide comfort and nutrition tailored to their stage.

While assigning a breast to each child can work well for some, others prefer to alternate between sides, particularly if one breast produces significantly more milk than the other. This is not necessarily a problem unless it bothers you.

- **Both breasts for both children:** Allowing both children to nurse from both breasts can ensure both are fully emptied, stimulating milk production and preventing engorgement.

- **Both children at different times:** Nursing separately can make sessions feel less overwhelming and give you a chance to connect with each child individually.

- **Both children at the same time:** Feeding both children simultaneously can save time and create a shared bonding experience. It may require experimenting with different positions to find what works best for you.

Stopping Tandem Nursing

You may decide to allow your children to nurse to term, meaning each child continues until they naturally self-wean. However, if you choose to stop breastfeeding one or both children before self-weaning, that's perfectly okay too.

When weaning an older child, focus on the positives – emphasise their 'big kid' privileges and reassure them of your continued love and connection. Redirect them with alternatives like a special cuddle or a favourite activity. Comfort them and let them know that you're not going anywhere, even if your breastfeeding journey is coming to an end. I discuss this stage of breastfeeding at length in the next chapter of this book (see page 265).

Breastfeeding while pregnant, and tandem feeding are remarkable feats of love and adaptability. Both require patience, creativity and a deep well of compassion – not only for your children but also for yourself. Whatever approach you take, remember that your path is uniquely yours. Celebrate the connections you're building and the care you're pouring into your family, and always remember that you are doing an *extraordinary* job.

CHAPTER TEN

How to Stop Breastfeeding

I consider parent-led weaning to be my speciality. Why? Because as the mother of a neurodivergent, bona fide boob-monster with a passion for gentle and responsive parenting, our weaning journey was hard-fought! It required meticulous planning, patience, consistency and a lot of self-reflection.

I wholeheartedly believe that every mother should be empowered to breastfeed on her own terms. For my friend Naomi, that meant nursing all three of her children until they allowed themselves to self-wean. Two of them did this at 4 years old, and her youngest is still nursing at 3 years old as I write this book. That has meant that she has been nursing for over seven years to date, with no end in sight. However, for many of the mothers I work with, they are ready to move away from breastfeeding much sooner than that.

For some mothers, weaning happens naturally over time, while for others, it requires careful planning, patience and emotional preparation. Some may choose to stop breastfeeding earlier than they initially expected due to returning to work, personal well-being, medical reasons or simply feeling ready to move on.

Take, for example, my client Sophie, who decided to wean her nine-month-old daughter, Isla. Sophie loved nursing but found herself physically and emotionally drained from the demands that night nursing, in particular, placed upon her body and mind. After months of exhaustion and struggling to find balance, she knew it was time to make a change. With a gradual approach – offering alternative comfort measures, introducing a bedtime routine that didn't rely on nursing and enlisting her partner's support – she was able to wean Isla in a way that felt gentle and responsive while also honouring her own needs.

This chapter will explore different approaches to weaning, from gentle, gradual transitions to more structured approaches, while addressing common challenges such as emotional attachment, night weaning and managing engorgement. Whatever your reasons for weaning, this chapter will help you feel confident, informed and supported as you navigate this next stage of your breastfeeding journey.

Our Weaning Story

I used to wonder what people meant when they talked about feeling 'touched out'. I had been back at work since my boy was around nine months old and I always looked forward to rushing home to nurse him. But by the time we were approaching three years of breastfeeding, things started to shift.

I was still nursing on demand, but something had changed. Was it because my son was much bigger physically? Or perhaps I was craving more space and time for myself? Whatever the reason, I began to feel frustrated and resentful when he asked to 'Boob'. I'd read about breastfeeding aversion being common around a mother's menstrual cycle, so initially, I thought it was just that.

I spent some time journalling and reflecting and I realised that I was happy to nurse my son first thing in the morning and overnight, but during the day, I needed some respite. I hadn't realised until then that I needed to give myself permission to wean – guilt-free. So, I decided to implement some boundaries during the day. I started having conversations with him about how one day, when he was bigger, all the milk would be in his belly and none left in my boobs. My tone was light, but his reaction was visceral, and I felt deeply guilty for causing him any distress.

Over the next weeks, I continued to introduce boundaries, saying 'No baby, not now' when he asked to nurse at various points throughout the day. Some days this led to whimpers and pawing at my top, other days it led to full-blown meltdowns. Gradually, the frequency of these became less and less and our new routine of nursing just twice a day and during overnight wake-ups began. For a month or so, this felt manageable and even enjoyable, but soon, the old feelings returned. My son would nurse to sleep and my skin would crawl. Why was this happening? Was my body done with giving so much of myself? What about my goal of natural term weaning?

Ultimately, I decided to wean my son after a bout of illness. We were both physically and mentally exhausted, and I was struggling to cope with his increased clinginess. He had previously been sleeping through the night, but after getting sick, he clung to me day and night and the more he clung, the more I felt like running the other way. One night, I broke. 'I can't do this,' I whispered to my fiancé, between sobs. 'I can't do this.' He took our son downstairs, screaming his heart out, while I buried my head under the covers.

I felt incredibly guilty that things had gotten to the stage of me being at breaking point before I had set clearer, more loving boundaries. It was only in hindsight that I realised it was my lack of boundaries and my fear of introducing them that had led to the situation. My son could feel my anxiety and apprehension about weaning, and as his mother, he needed me to take the lead and guide him through this process. So, I began to put together a plan.

This is the strategy I used and use with my clients. Over the next few months, I dropped the morning feed, kept communication open with him and started introducing comfort associations. Slowly, I began limiting his bedtime and overnight feeds too. After a while, he was only nursing for a minute before being rocked to sleep by me or his dad.

At one point, I wondered if it was actually me who was clinging to those last moments before bed, rather than him. During the last few weeks of breastfeeding my mood began to plummet. I felt like I was living in a haze, with my emotions all over the place, my tears frequent. I was plagued with nightmares and nausea, and I questioned my decision to wean every day. But sure enough, every time my son nursed to sleep, I felt my teeth clenching through the discomfort. I was ready to stop completely – I just needed to get through the weaning blues.

A week before our last feed, I suggested to my son that we choose a date for his 'last boob'. I expected a tantrum, but was completely taken aback when he said, 'Okay, how about tomorrow?' My eyes welled up, and I squeezed him tight. He was ready, but was I? In the end, my son nursed one more time after his 'last feed', in the middle of the night after my fiancé and I had been out for a Valentine's date. I absentmindedly allowed him to latch, thinking nothing of it. Part of me wishes I'd known it would be the last time, but another part of me is glad it was so natural and gradual.

My weaning blues lasted about eight weeks, but they eventually subsided after we stopped breastfeeding. Introducing boundaries took much more from me than I anticipated, but I'm glad I did it. I wish I had introduced them sooner, before reaching breaking point. Perhaps I needed to reach that point to feel confident about my decision, but I realise now that, just like at the start of breastfeeding, I needed someone who had been there to guide me through every step.

Weaning Blues: Understanding the Hormonal Shift

Many mothers are caught off-guard by the emotional impact of weaning, often referred to as weaning blues. While stopping breastfeeding is a natural transition, it triggers a significant hormonal shift that can affect both your mood and overall well-being.

Why Do Weaning Blues Happen?

During breastfeeding, your body produces oxytocin and prolactin, hormones that not only support milk production but also promote feelings of relaxation, calm and connection. When breastfeeding stops, these hormone levels drop, creating a temporary hormonal imbalance before your body gradually returns to its pre-lactation state.

This hormonal watershed can lead to:

- **Mood changes**, including irritability, anxiety or feelings of sadness.

- **Insomnia or vivid dreams**, as oxytocin levels decrease (oxytocin helps to regulate sleep).

- **Physical symptoms** like headaches, hot flashes, nausea or fatigue.

- **A sense of loss or grief**, especially if breastfeeding was a deeply emotional experience.

The Link Between Weaning and Postnatal Depression

Research suggests that abrupt or unplanned weaning may increase the risk of postnatal depression (PND).

This is because the sudden drop in prolactin and oxytocin can leave mothers feeling depleted, particularly if they are already vulnerable to mood fluctuations. While not every mother will experience these effects, it's important to be aware that weaning can be an emotionally challenging time – and that these feelings are valid and temporary.

Understanding why these emotional and physical shifts occur can help you prepare for them rather than feeling blindsided. Just as your body adapted to breastfeeding, it will adjust to weaning – but it takes time. Knowing what to expect can help you make informed choices, whether that means weaning gradually, seeking additional support or practising self-care strategies to help stabilise mood and energy levels.

While I discuss the hormonal impact of weaning more in-depth later in this chapter, I want to emphasise here that if you are struggling, you are not alone. The emotional weight of weaning is real, and seeking support – whether from loved ones, a healthcare professional or a supportive community – can make all the difference.

Child-led Weaning

Child-led weaning is a gradual and natural process where your baby or toddler decides when they are ready to stop breastfeeding. It's a journey that honours your child's needs and timing while respecting your own feelings and boundaries. This typically happens when your little one shows signs of independence and a decreasing interest in nursing. You might notice that they start to reduce the frequency of nursing sessions or become more interested in food, toys or other activities instead of breastfeeding.

For some babies, weaning may happen naturally as they become more independent or grow into their own comfort mechanisms. For others, the process can be a slow, tender transition that may require gentle encouragement. In either case, it's important to stay in tune with your baby's readiness and respect their cues. They may not seem as eager to nurse during the day but still want that closeness at night. It's about recognising that weaning isn't something that happens all at once, but in small steps, based on your child's developmental pace. It's crucial to remain patient and flexible throughout, and trust that your child will guide you as you both navigate this change together.

Parent-led Weaning

Parent-led weaning is when you, as a parent, make the decision to stop breastfeeding. Whether that's due to personal choice, returning to work or any other reason. This method gives you control over the process, but it still requires gentleness and respect for your child's emotions. If you are ready to begin weaning, it's important to approach it with the same care and empathy that you've used throughout your breastfeeding journey.

The key to successful parent-led weaning is clear communication, setting gentle boundaries and recognising that this process will take time. When you decide that it's time to stop breastfeeding, it's important to gradually reduce the number of feeds rather than stopping suddenly. This gradual approach helps your child adjust emotionally, while also allowing your body to adapt to a decreased demand for milk. Parent-led weaning can be empowering because it allows you to take control of your own timeline, but remember, it's still a process that requires sensitivity as it may bring up strong feelings for both you and your child. I break this down step by step later in this chapter, but first, let's explore some common weaning practices that I do not recommend.

Don't Expect a Weekend Away to Work

While some people might suggest taking a weekend away to 'force' the weaning process, I cannot recommend this approach. While it may seem like a quick solution, it can often be disruptive for both you and your child. Abrupt weaning, especially if your body has been producing milk on demand, can be physically painful, leading to engorgement, clogged ducts or even mastitis. Moreover, this approach doesn't give your child a chance to process the transition in a gentle way. Imagine if your partner suddenly stopped showing you affection without any explanation; you'd be left feeling confused and hurt. It's the same for your child when breastfeeding suddenly stops without a clear, loving conversation.

Weaning is a process that can be done with intention, patience and respect for both your body and your child's emotional needs. While it can be tempting to try to avoid the discomfort of the transition, giving yourself time to gradually reduce the breastfeeding sessions and build new comforting habits with your child is the gentlest approach.

Don't Lead with Distraction

Another common piece of advice I hear is to distract your child whenever they want to nurse. While it's true that focussing their attention elsewhere can sometimes help in moments of frustration, leading with distraction can leave your child feeling confused and unsettled. This tactic doesn't provide the emotional clarity or reassurance your child needs. Putting the onus on distraction, rather than addressing the underlying emotional need for connection could inadvertently lead to more anxiety for your little one.

Instead of using distraction as a primary tool, I recommend using it as one part of a broader, more empathetic strategy. As your child begins to understand the changes around breastfeeding, offering comforting alternatives, like reading a story or cuddling, can help them navigate the transition without confusion. The key here is to approach weaning with patience and understanding – creating a new routine that feels both secure and gentle for them.

Don't Seek Perfection

This is something I've had to remind myself of constantly during this journey: weaning, like all aspects of parenting, is not about perfection. There will be days when things go smoothly, and others when you feel like you're not making any progress at all. Some days, you'll experience moments of doubt or guilt. You might wonder if you're doing the right thing or if you're somehow failing. But remember this – there is no correct way to wean, and there is no 'right' timeline for every family. The journey is unique to you and your child, and that's what makes it beautiful.

Perfectionism can be a major obstacle to navigating this transition smoothly. Instead of striving for flawless execution, focus on the progress, the small wins and the ways you and your child are learning and growing together. Allow space for mistakes, reflect on how you can improve and embrace the process. Weaning is a learning curve and it's okay to take it one step at a time.

Do Expect Weaning to Be a Process

Weaning is not an overnight event – it's a process that evolves over time. Just like any major transition in life, it takes time, patience and often some adjustments along the way. For many families, weaning can take months and it may feel like a slow and gradual process of introducing boundaries, comfort and new routines. Some children will self-wean naturally, while others might need more time and encouragement to let go of breastfeeding. The timeline is different for everyone, and that's completely okay.

There may be times when you feel like you're taking two steps forward and one step back. Your child might seem ready one day and then ask for 'boob' the next. That's perfectly normal. As you introduce new boundaries, the process may feel messy and imperfect and that's part of what makes it real and beautiful. Expect bumps along the way, but rest assured that the consistency of your approach will lead to positive results over time.

Gentle Weaning: Nourishing and Supporting Young Babies and Toddlers Through the Process

Weaning is a deeply personal and emotional transition, and whether your child is a few months old or a toddler, the process requires compassion, patience and gradual adjustment. The following steps outline a gentle and responsive approach that can work for both younger and older babies, ensuring that the transition feels supported and secure.

Step One: Permission to Wean

Before anything else, you need to give yourself permission to stop breastfeeding. This is a big, emotional decision and it's important to accept that you're choosing to end this chapter of your nursing journey on your terms. Let go of any guilt or pressure from outside influences and focus on what's best for both you and your little one.

For mothers of younger babies who may not have intended to wean so soon, this step can feel particularly difficult. If you are stopping for medical, emotional or logistical reasons, it's normal to experience feelings of grief alongside relief. Your decision to wean does not diminish the love, care or connection you share with your baby.

Step Two: Communicate with Your Child

For toddlers and older babies, communication is key. Even if they don't fully understand, talking about the transition can be reassuring. Use simple, calm phrases like, 'Milk will be all-gone soon,' and 'We can cuddle instead.' A really beautiful way to communicate this is by explaining that soon your milk will be 'all-gone' from your boobs, but that it's in your little one's heart, bones and skin forever. Role-playing or showing what bedtime will look like without breastfeeding can also help ease the transition.

For younger babies (under 12 months) who do not yet understand words, communication happens through consistent, loving reassurance. Since they rely on the physical act of nursing for comfort, you can support the transition by maintaining gentle physical closeness, skin-to-skin contact and responding promptly to their cues. While they may not understand language, they will feel the security of your presence, helping them adjust to the change.

Step Three: Layer Comfort Associations/Habit Stacking

This step is about introducing new comfort mechanisms alongside breastfeeding, so the transition away from nursing feels gradual and reassuring. I recommend adding in at least three more comfort or sleep associations alongside nursing and give them time to take hold before you move on to step four. For some babies this happens as quickly as just a few days, whereas it may take weeks or even months for others.

- For toddlers, you might introduce rocking, singing or a bedtime story as new comfort associations.
- For younger babies, alternative soothing methods like gentle swaying, rhythmic patting, white noise or pacifiers

can help meet their natural need for sucking and closeness. Babywearing or contact napping can also provide security in place of nursing.

If you can layer these new associations *before* you start moving away from breastfeeding, you will help your child feel supported rather than abruptly losing a source of comfort.

A Sleep Story

A sleep story is a made-up story which you reserve specifically for bedtimes. It lasts for 5–10 minutes and – as far as possible – you tell it to your child every time they are about to go to sleep. Make the story about you and the people your child loves. It should involve you all doing everyday things or going on an adventure – perhaps changing the story slightly every night. The point is to keep your child listening to your reassuring voice until they drift off. Include some of their favourite things to keep it engaging, but try not to make it too exciting and stimulating.

Below is an example of the start of a story which I told my son for months at a time when we were making the transition to stopping nursing to sleep. It is inspired by the time that I spent living in Abu Dhabi – a place we have not yet visited as a family, but my son has heard me talk about often:

One day, mummy, daddy and baby (use your child(ren)'s name) were off on an adventure. They headed to Birmingham airport in a shiny black taxi, ready to board a plane to take them to Abu Dhabi. It was sunrise when they arrived at the airport and the sky was painted pink,

> *lilac and coral. Mummy, daddy and baby went through airport security, checked in their luggage and headed to the terminal. It was a busy morning, with people hustling and bustling to and fro. When they arrived at the terminal, they spotted the huge airbus A380 (my son loves aeroplanes!) ready to take them to the desert.*
>
> *They settled into their seats on the plane, with the baby sitting closest to the window. He watched the cars and buildings below disappear into the clouds as we ascended in the huge metal bird. The turbine engines hummed as we glided above the city and then the ocean and mountains, until we were in the Middle East. Slowly, the plane descended, gliding through the clouds once more until we landed with a gentle bump on the tarmac at Abu Dhabi airport...*
>
> You could even record yourself saying this story on your phone or another device so that it can be played in your absence – on repeat!

Step Four: Introduce a Boundary

Once you feel confident in your decision, introduce a gentle boundary. This step can be adapted based on your baby's age and temperament:

- For older babies and toddlers, you might say, 'Not now, we'll nurse at bedtime,' comfort them and redirect them to another activity.

- For younger babies, since verbal reasoning isn't possible, spacing out feeds slightly, offering extra cuddles or changing feeding positions can help gradually shift the pattern of nursing without causing them unnecessary distress.

- Introduce bottles gradually – If possible, start by replacing one breastfeeding session at a time with a bottle of donor milk or formula, allowing your baby time to adjust.

- Mix breast milk with formula – To help your baby get used to the taste and texture of formula, prepare the formula first according to the instructions on the package. **Never add dry formula directly to breast milk, as this can be dangerous.** Once the formula is properly mixed, you can add breast milk in **decreasing** amounts over time. Gradually, you can replace the breast milk with more formula, so that the bottle becomes mostly formula as your baby adjusts.

- Use paced bottle feeding (see Chapter Eight page 233). Hold your baby in your arms and allow them to control the flow of milk to mimic breastfeeding. This can help prevent overfeeding and make the transition smoother.

The key is to remain consistent and calm. Your baby or toddler will likely express frustration and that's okay. Change is hard, but your loving presence will help them adjust, just as it will at other major transitions in their life.

Step Five: Increase the Boundary

Once initial boundaries are in place, gradually reduce nursing duration and frequency:

- For toddlers, shorten nursing sessions by counting down ('We'll do ten sips, then all done') or slowly replace feeds with another activity.

- For younger babies, you may start offering a bottle, cup or alternative soothing method first before breastfeeding, helping them adjust to a different feeding experience.

- Encourage a variety of nutrient-dense foods – Focus on protein, healthy fats and iron-rich foods, ensuring they get enough energy throughout the day.

- For 6–12-month-olds, offer solids before dropping multiple feeds. Your baby will naturally increase their solid intake over time, but milk should still make up around 500–600ml (16–20oz) per day during this stage.

- Introduce little sips of water – babies can start drinking small amounts of water beyond six months (from an open cup, sippy cup or straw cup) alongside meals to support their hydration.

At this stage, some children naturally lose interest and stop asking to nurse. Others may need more reassurance and time, which is completely normal. Trust that your baby or toddler will find new ways to feel secure and you will find new ways to connect.

Step Six: Preparing for an Emotional Transition

Once you have established boundaries, take a moment to reflect on your journey. Weaning is not just a change for your child – it's a major shift for you, too. Whether you are weaning at six months or after several years, you deserve to recognise and honour your breastfeeding experience.

Would you like to celebrate with a keepsake, write a letter to your child about your journey or simply take a moment to reflect on the bond you've shared? However you choose to close this chapter, remember: your love and care continue far beyond breastfeeding.

Step Seven: Your Last Feed

When the time comes for the last feed, it may feel bittersweet. You've both shared so many beautiful moments through breastfeeding, and now you're entering a new phase. Take time to savour the final feed, whether it's expected or spontaneous. If your child is ready, it will be a gentle and natural transition, one that marks the end of this chapter and the beginning of another.

Remember, this is your journey, and you've done an incredible job nurturing your child. Be kind to yourself as you navigate this next phase and know that you are not alone in this process. Weaning can be an emotional transition, but it doesn't have to feel like a loss. Your baby or toddler will continue to thrive with love, nourishment and new routines, even as breastfeeding comes to an end. Trust that they will adapt and so will you.

Whether your journey lasted six weeks, six months or several years, your decision to wean with love and care is something to be proud of. You are still your baby's source of comfort, security and connection – no matter how they are fed.

Navigating the Emotional Transition of Stopping Breastfeeding

When you decide to stop breastfeeding, it's important to recognise the significant hormonal shifts that accompany this huge emotional and physical transition. Just as during pregnancy or menopause, ceasing breastfeeding triggers a decrease in oxytocin and prolactin – the main hormones responsible for milk production. Beyond their role in breastfeeding, these hormones contribute to feelings of calm and happiness for as long as you are nursing or pumping.

However, when you stop breastfeeding, it takes time for your body to adjust and your other feel-good hormones will slowly return to their natural balance. This temporary hormonal gap can bring on various symptoms such as insomnia, brain fog, irritability, low mood and tearfulness. Some women also experience physical symptoms like hot flushes, headaches or nausea, as well as an overwhelming sense of grief that can accompany this process.

Every woman's experience with these hormonal fluctuations is unique. Some may find the transition smoother, while others may feel more affected. It's also worth noting that older mothers, in particular, may be more susceptible to weaning depression due to their stage in the oestrogen life cycle. That is to say that over your lifetime, your oestrogen levels gradually decline. Therefore, if you're an older mother who has been nursing for years, you will likely be later along your unique oestrogen cycle and more likely to notice feeling different once you stop lactating.

When I weaned my son at three years and nine months, I was ready, yet not prepared for how emotionally challenging it would be. Despite planning, reflecting and gradually introducing boundaries, I was still struck by waves of grief as we approached our final feed. As someone who had worked with many mothers and understood the science behind what are sometimes known as 'weaning blues', I still found myself caught off-guard. While I was relieved that our nursing and pumping journey was over, I also found myself swimming in the depths of grief. I felt as though I spent my days wading through a dense fog which obscured the beauty in life. Insomnia and nightmares plagued my nights, which felt like a cruel irony since my son had only started sleeping longer stretches that previous year. I also experienced waves of nausea, headaches, hot flushes, brain fog and low motivation. It was a depression in every sense of the word and it was a month or two before the clouds started to lift and I began to feel brighter.

If you're struggling with weaning depression, please know that you're not alone. It's entirely normal to feel a mixture of emotions and a range of physical effects during this time.

Below are some compassionate and realistic strategies that will help you weather this transition:

1. **Stabilise Your Blood Sugar Levels**
   Make sure to eat protein-rich meals and snacks throughout the day. This helps support stable energy levels, and in turn can reduce feelings of irritability and low mood.

2. **Stay Hydrated**
   Prioritising hydration is key, especially as your body adjusts. Carry a water bottle with you and keep a glass of water beside your bed so you can sip it first thing in the morning. Staying hydrated can also help with mood swings and physical symptoms like headaches.

3. **Get Outdoors**
   Aim for at least 30 minutes outside each day, preferably in natural surroundings and sunlight. This could be as simple as eating your lunch at a local park rather than at home or at your desk. Or you could take your little one for a stroll after dinner but before bedtime. However you do it, spending time outdoors can improve your mood and enhance the quality of your sleep, helping you feel more grounded.

4. **Incorporate Kefir-based Products into your Diet**
   Some studies suggest that kefir-based yoghurts and drinks may have a positive effect on mood, potentially reducing depressive symptoms. These probiotics can also support gut health, which plays an important role in mental health.

5. **Journalling for Self-reflection**
   Journalling can be an incredibly healing way to process your emotions during this time. Set aside a few minutes each day to reflect on how you're feeling. Use the following prompts to guide your thoughts:
   - How do I feel about no longer breastfeeding?
   - What has been the most challenging part of the day for me during this transition?
   - What do I miss the most about breastfeeding?
   - Who can I turn to for support during this time?
   - What activities or habits help me cope?
   - What is my favourite memory of breastfeeding?
   - What do I need more or less of at the moment?
   - How can I show more compassion towards myself as I navigate this process?
   - What permissions can I grant myself during this transition?

It's common for weaning blues to persist for up to eight weeks, but if after a month or so you don't start to feel any better, please consider reaching out for additional support. This could be from a healthcare professional, a naturopath or a hormone specialist. Remember, you deserve just as much care, grace and love at the end of your breastfeeding journey as you did at the beginning. With the right support, these difficult feelings will eventually ease and brighter days will come. You deserve to feel supported, confident and empowered as you transition through weaning. Take your time, be kind to yourself and trust in your own strength and resilience throughout this process.

CHAPTER ELEVEN

Celebrating Your Breastfeeding Journey

Breastfeeding is a profound and transformative experience. It's an emotional, physical and spiritual journey that connects you to your baby in ways words often fail to express. The bond shared through breastfeeding is unlike any other, one that deepens over time, with each feed creating an intricate web of love, comfort and closeness. In this chapter, we celebrate that journey. We honour the months and years of breastfeeding, recognising that it is not always easy, but it is always meaningful. Regardless of how long your breastfeeding journey has lasted or even if it is still ongoing, it is worthy of celebration. The challenges you've faced, the growth you've experienced, and the love you've shared all come together in this special time. Let's take a moment to reflect, celebrate and empower you as you continue to nurture your little one beyond breastfeeding.

Honouring Every Breastfeeding Journey

Breastfeeding takes many forms, and every journey is deeply personal. For some mothers, it lasts just a few days or weeks, while others continue for months or even years. No matter how long you breastfeed, whether for a short season or well into toddlerhood, your effort and dedication deserve recognition. The beauty of breastfeeding lies not in its duration but in the love, care, and connection it fosters between you and your child.

The reality is that breastfeeding can look different for everyone. Some mothers exclusively breastfeed, others combination-feed, pump or use donor milk. Some transition to formula when it becomes the right choice for their family. Regardless of the path taken, what remains constant is the devotion to nurturing and sustaining a growing baby in the best way possible for both mother and child.

Weaning Ceremonies and Traditions

For many cultures around the world, the end of breastfeeding has been marked by special ceremonies, recognising the milestone in a way that honours both mother and child. These ceremonies can provide a meaningful way to celebrate the end of this phase, while also providing support during what can sometimes be a challenging transition. Here are two examples of weaning traditions that may inspire you as you navigate this period:

- Breast milk jewellery is made by carefully preserving your breast milk and setting the preserved milk into a piece of jewellery – typically a pendant, ring or earrings. You can buy DIY kits for making your own jewellery, but if you can, I recommend having it professionally made. To do this, find a maker that you like online and send them a small amount of your milk to preserve in a jewellery design of your choice.

- A nursing photo shoot, a boob party (complete with boob-shaped cake) or even a ceremony to commemorate your journey.

Weaning Ceremonies Around the World

1. The 'First Feed' Ceremony

In South Africa, some families celebrate the introduction of solid foods with a ceremony known as the 'First Feed'. This event acknowledges the shift from exclusive breastfeeding to incorporating solids, a moment when the child begins to explore a broader world of nourishment. The ceremony often involves the family and community gathering, offering blessings and expressing gratitude for the mother's dedication to breastfeeding. It is a time to celebrate the child's growth and the mother's role in nurturing them, marking the beginning of a new chapter while recognising the importance of the breastfeeding journey.

2. The Weaning Ceremony

In Mali, West Africa, a 'weaning ceremony' is held to celebrate a child's transition from breastfeeding to eating solid foods. This marks a significant milestone in the child's development. The event typically involves a gathering of family and friends, where the child is presented with new foods. It is a moment of joy and reflection, as both mother and child are supported in this new phase of growth. This ceremony not only celebrates the child's increased independence but also acknowledges the mother's role in nurturing and nourishing her child.

3. The Weaning Ritual

In Ancient Rome there was a formal ritual surrounding the weaning process, usually when the child reached two or three years old. This ritual, while less formalised than modern ceremonies, often involved symbolic acts such as presenting the child with new clothing or items that marked their transition from infancy to childhood. The ritual was a way of recognising the shift in the mother-child relationship as the child moved away from the breast, but it also honoured the close bond created through breastfeeding.

Incorporating a ceremonial approach to weaning can offer both mothers and children a meaningful way to transition. This chapter of your journey may come to an end, but the memories and connection you've built with your child will last forever.

The Impact of Breastfeeding – In Any Form

Every drop of breast milk matters for your baby. Breast milk contains antibodies that support a baby's immune system, essential nutrients that promote growth and hormones that help with bonding and comfort. But beyond its nutritional benefits breastfeeding also represents the care, patience and sacrifice that mothers make every single day.

For mothers who breastfeed into toddlerhood and beyond, the benefits continue to evolve. Breastfeeding at this stage becomes more about comfort, emotional regulation and connection rather than just nutrition. It weaves itself into everyday life, providing reassurance during big transitions and a moment of stillness in the chaos of early childhood. However, just as extended breastfeeding has its joys, it also comes with challenges – whether navigating societal expectations, balancing personal needs or managing the gradual weaning process.

At the same time, for mothers who transition away from breastfeeding earlier, the love and connection they share with their child are just as profound. Weaning can be bittersweet, whether it happens sooner than expected or exactly as planned. What matters most is that we as mothers feel confident in our choices, knowing that our bond with our children remains strong, regardless of how our feeding journey unfolded.

Celebrating Every Mother's Choice

Breastfeeding – whether for a few weeks or several years – requires patience, resilience and immense love. Some mothers stop breastfeeding because they feel ready, others because of external circumstances beyond their control. Some never planned to breastfeed, while others grieve when their journey ends earlier than expected. Every experience is valid and every mother deserves to be celebrated for the ways she nourishes and nurtures her child.

If you are still breastfeeding, know that your journey is unique and your experience is yours to define. If you have weaned, remember that the connection you've built with your child extends far beyond breastfeeding. However you have fed your baby, you have provided for them in ways that only you could.

Most importantly, know that you are not alone. No matter what stage you are in, there is a community of mothers who understand, support and celebrate you. Whether you are breastfeeding, weaning or have already moved on to the next chapter, you are doing an incredible job. Each of our journeys are different, but everyone is worth honouring.

Words of Wisdom and Affirmations

As you reflect on your breastfeeding journey, remember that you have given your child everything they need – nourishment, comfort, security and above all, your unwavering love. There is no one 'right' way to feed your child. Whether you breastfed for a few months or a few years, your experience is uniquely yours and deserves to be celebrated.

Here are some affirmations to carry with you as you conclude your breastfeeding journey:

- *I have made the best choice for my child and for me.*
- *I am confident in my ability to nourish and care for my child, regardless of what others may say.*
- *My bond with my child is unbreakable and breastfeeding has strengthened it in ways I never imagined.*
- *I am proud of how far I have come and how much I have given.*
- *I honour my body for the work it has done for our family.*

You, dear mama, have nourished, nurtured and loved your child through breastfeeding. This chapter may be closing, but the foundation of love, trust and connection you've built with your little one will stay with you both forever. And that's something to be celebrated, now and always.

It's okay to acknowledge the emotions that come with weaning or transitioning to a new phase. It's also okay to feel a sense of loss, but remember that you have given your child the very best start. Trust in yourself and take pride in the love you've shared.

A Love Letter

Writing a letter to yourself can be a powerful way to reflect on your breastfeeding journey, celebrate the milestones you've reached and acknowledge the challenges you've faced. This letter allows you to process your thoughts and emotions, creating a beautiful memento of this significant part of your life.

Here's a guide to help you write your own personal letter.

1. **Start with Your Journey to Motherhood**

Begin by reflecting on the journey that led you to become a mother. Consider the events that brought you to this point. Think about the moment you found out you were pregnant and the emotions that arose from that news. Reflect on your pregnancy and the birth of your baby – acknowledge how incredible you are for bringing your baby into the world. Even if the path wasn't smooth, you were strong and capable in your journey.

2. **Reflect on Your Postpartum Experience**

Shift your focus to the postpartum journey – the moment you first met your baby and how your relationship grew. Think about the special moments of bonding that you shared with your baby. What were the things you did that made you feel proud of yourself? There are moments that may have felt difficult or uncertain – be gentle with yourself and acknowledge them. Recognise what you've done well and also what you might not have given yourself credit for. This is an opportunity to affirm the strength you've shown.

3. **Focus on Your Nursing or Pumping Journey**

Now, reflect on your breastfeeding or pumping experience. How did breastfeeding or pumping evolve for you? What were the challenges and triumphs? What did you learn about yourself through this process? Whether you were able to nurse as long as you wanted or had to navigate other ways of providing nourishment, remember that you have given so much, you have done your best and your efforts have mattered.

4. Look Ahead to Your Motherhood Journey

Take a moment to think about the next chapter in your motherhood journey. Breastfeeding has been such a significant part of your experience, but now it's time to look ahead to all the other beautiful, messy and meaningful moments that await. What kind of relationship do you hope to continue to build with your child as they grow? Reflect on the ways in which you've nurtured them so far and the ways you can continue to nurture them – whether through shared adventures, moments of comfort or fostering independence.

Remember, you are more than a breastfeeding mother and your bond with your child goes beyond this one aspect of your relationship. Think about your hopes for the future: what kind of parent do you want to be as your child enters new phases of life? Whether you're supporting them through early milestones or guiding them as they grow into their own person, your role as a mother continues to evolve.

Here is the letter I wrote to myself at the end of our nursing journey. It was an incredibly emotional and cathartic process and as I re-read it years later, it fills me with pride and gratitude for all that I did and gave to our precious rainbow baby boy. I hope that it inspires your own:

> *Dear Me,*
>
> *As you close the chapter on this incredible breastfeeding journey, take a moment to truly see and honour the depth of your devotion. For three years and nine months, you*

gave of yourself completely – morning, noon and night – out of pure love and a fierce commitment to your son's health, well-being and happiness. The energy, effort and time you poured into nourishing him came from a place so selfless that you didn't even fully recognise the weight of what you were carrying until you finally laid it down. Every late-night feed, every moment spent soothing, every millilitre of milk shared was a testament to your profound dedication. You sacrificed comfort, sleep and so much of yourself to give him the best start in life, and that is something extraordinary.

This journey was not without its challenges, yet you persevered. You faced thrush, bleeding nipples and the exhaustion of oversupply. You navigated the strain of reflux and endured a lack of support from friends, family and colleagues. Yet you never gave up. Through every trial, you found the strength to keep going, driven by your love for your son and your belief in the bond you were building. And what a bond it is – a connection rooted in trust, love and nourishment that will last a lifetime. The health benefits you gifted him through your persistence are priceless, extending far beyond the days of nursing. In every way, you overcame the impossible and showed a resilience that deserves to be celebrated.

Now, as you move forward in your motherhood journey, carry with you the legacy of love you created during these years. The time, energy and care you invested in breastfeeding were never just about milk; they were about showing your son, in every moment, that he is cherished. That legacy will continue to shape him long after your nursing days are behind you. And let this be a reminder to yourself: You have done something remarkable. You are still doing remarkable things every single day. Motherhood is not about perfection, but about love – and you have given that love in abundance.

So, as you close this chapter and look towards the future, give yourself the credit and grace you deserve. Know that the love you poured into your son during this journey will echo through his life and yours in ways you may not even fully see yet. Be proud, Mama – you gave your all, and it was more than enough.

With love and deep admiration,
Myself

Reflective Journalling and Meditation

As you now reflect on your journey as a mother, I invite you to pause and look inward. Take a moment to consider the power of your choices, the strength of your love and the wisdom you've gathered. Reflect on how far you've come and how beautifully your relationship with your child has evolved. This time is for you to embrace yourself with love, understanding and acceptance. Use the following prompts and meditations to empower your heart and mind, as you continue your journey with confidence and grace.

Journal Prompts

1. **Reflecting on Your Journey:**

    o   What are three moments from your breastfeeding or parenting journey that stand out to you as particularly meaningful? Why do these moments hold such significance for you?

    o   What have you learned about yourself through the process of motherhood so far? How have you grown as a person, as a mother and as an individual?

2. **Empowerment in Choice:**
   - How has making choices that align with your values and circumstances shaped your motherhood? How do you feel when you think about the power you have to make decisions on your own terms?
   - What are some choices you are most proud of, no matter how small or big they may seem?

3. **Unconditional Love for Yourself:**
   - In what ways can you show yourself the same compassion and care that you offer to your child? What do you need to hear today to affirm your worth as a mother and as a person?
   - Write a letter to yourself from a place of unconditional love. What would your heart tell you if it could speak freely and without judgment?

4. **Moving Forward with Confidence:**
   - What does motherhood on *your* terms look like as you move forward? How does it feel to honour your needs, desires and well-being alongside your child's?
   - Imagine your future self as a mother. What do you want to remember about this moment and what advice would your future self give to you today?

5. **Acknowledging the Transformative Power of Motherhood:**
   - How has your relationship with your child evolved over time? How do you anticipate that evolving connection will look as they grow older? What

hopes do you have for the next stage of your motherhood journey?
   - What role does joy play in your relationship with your child? How can you intentionally cultivate more moments of joy in your everyday interactions?

6. **Affirmations for Moving Forward:**
   - Write a list of affirmations that empower you in your motherhood journey. What affirmations resonate with your soul, reminding you that you are doing enough and that you are worthy of love, care and peace?

Final Thoughts

As you reach the final pages of *The Breastfeeding Survival Guide*, I hope you feel a deep sense of empowerment and connection to your own journey. This book was never intended to provide a one-size-fits-all formula for motherhood or breastfeeding. Instead, it has been designed as a supportive companion to help you navigate the myriad paths that can unfold in your role as a mother.

The truth is, every mother has everything she needs within her to mother authentically and intuitively. You are the expert on your child, on your family and on your life. Trusting your instincts, listening to your body and honouring your unique journey is at the heart of being a mother.

Motherhood can feel isolating at times, especially in a world that often expects us to go it alone, to be self-sufficient and unshaken. The reality is that parenting, like breastfeeding, is a communal experience. You don't have to face it all in solitude. We are all in this together – for all our sakes. It is through connection, community and open-hearted support that we find strength, wisdom and resilience.

The support you need can take many forms: whether it's a friend who listens without judgment, a breastfeeding counsellor who guides you with expertise or a group of mothers who remind you that they're in the same boat. These relationships are not only vital to your well-being, but they are what sustain the spirit of motherhood. When we come together, share our experiences and lift each other up, we honour the profound power of connection. This is where true empowerment lies: not in isolation, but in shared understanding and mutual care.

As you continue your breastfeeding journey or yours comes to an end, know that you are capable, resilient and deeply worthy of care. You are exactly the mother your child needs. And when challenges arise – because they will – you have the tools, knowledge and inner strength to meet them. Trust yourself, seek support when you need it and celebrate each small victory along the way.

If you remember nothing else from this book, I hope that you hold on to the truth that when we mothers thrive, the world thrives.

References

Introduction

CDC, 'Breastfeeding Report Card' (2022) https://www.cdc.gov/breastfeeding-data/breastfeeding-report-card/index.html

Alimi R., Azmoude E., Moradi M., Zamani M. The association of breastfeeding with a reduced risk of postpartum depression: a systematic review and meta-analysis. *Breastfeed Med.* 2022 Apr;17(4):268-278. doi: 10.1089/bfm.2021.0183.

House of Commons Health and Social Care Committee. Breastfeeding in the UK. Available from: https://www.unicef.org.uk/babyfriendly/about/breastfeeding-in-the-uk/.

Kendall-Tackett K., 'A new paradigm for depression in new mothers: The central role of inflammation and how breastfeeding and anti-inflammatory treatments protect maternal mental health'. *International Breastfeeding Journal.* 3(1) (2007): 17. https://internationalbreastfeedingjournal.biomedcentral.com/articles/10.1186/1746-4358-3-17

Morrison A.H., et al. Mothers' reasons for early breastfeeding cessation. Am J Maternal/Child Nursing. 2019;44(6):353–59. DOI: 10.1097/NMC.0000000000000580.

NHS Digital, 'Infant Feeding Survey 2010 – Early Results' (2011) https://digital.nhs.uk/data-and-information/publications/statistical/infant-feeding-survey/infant-feeding-survey-2010-early-results

Raphael D., *Being Female: Reproduction, Power and Change* (De Gruyter Mouton; 1975)

Slomian J., et al. Consequences of maternal postpartum depression: A systematic review of maternal and infant outcomes. *Women's Health.* 2019;15:1745506519844044. doi:10.1177/1745506519844044.

U.S. Centers for Disease Control and Prevention (CDC). Postpartum depression. https://www.cdc.gov/breastfeeding-special-circumstances/hcp/illnesses-conditions/postpartum-depression.html.

World Breastfeeding Trends Initiative (WBTi) UK. World Breastfeeding Trends Initiative (WBTi) UK Report 2024. UK Breastfeeding Foundation; March 2025.

World Health Organization (WHO). Breastfeeding. https://www.who.int/health-topics/breastfeeding#tab=tab_1

Chapter One: Beginning Breastfeeding

Azim H.A., et al. Breastfeeding in women with hormone receptor-positive breast cancer who conceived after temporary interruption of endocrine therapy: Results from the POSITIVE trial. Presented at ESMO Congress 2024.

Blondeaux E. et al, 'Breastfeeding after breast cancer in young BRCA carriers: results from an international cohort study'. Presented at ESMO Congress 2024.

Heinig M.J., Dewey K.G. Health effects of breastfeeding for mothers: a critical review. *Nutr Res Rev.* 1997 Jan;10(1):35–56. doi: 10.1079/NRR19970004. PMID: 19094257.

Jordan S.J., et al. Breastfeeding factors and risk of epithelial ovarian cancer. *J Clin Oncol.* 2019;37(4):319–327. Available from: PMC6558958.

Obeagu E.I., Obeagu G.U. Breastfeeding's protective role in alleviating breast cancer burden: a comprehensive review. *Breast Cancer.* 2023;29(4):789–795. PMCID: PMC11060284. PMID: 38694322.

The Nuffield Trust. Breastfeeding statistics in England. https://www.nuffieldtrust.org.uk/resource/breastfeeding

Unar-Munguía M., Torres-Mejía G., Colchero M.A., González de Cosío T. Breastfeeding and risk of breast cancer: A systematic review and meta-analysis. Acta Obstet Gynecol Scand. 2017;96(8):927–938. Available from: PMC10518059.

Chapter Three: Managing Your Milk Supply for Nursing and Pumping

Antenatal Training. Breastfeeding Counsellor Training. Available from: https://antenatal-training.com

Berens P., Eglash A., Malloy M., Steube A., Academy of Breastfeeding Medicine. ABM Clinical Protocol #26: Persistent Pain with Breastfeeding. Breastfeed Med. 2016;11(2):56–67. Available from: https://abm.memberclicks.net/assets/DOCUMENTS/PROTOCOLS/26-persistent-pain-protocol-english.pdf

Alabama Department of Public Health, 'Stomach Capacity' (2020). https://www.alabamapublichealth.gov/perinatal/assets/StomachCapacity.pdf

Cox D. B., Owens R. A., Hartmann P. E., 'Blood and milk prolactin and the rate of milk synthesis in women'. *Experimental Physiology* 81(6) (Nov, 1996): 1007–20.

Dewey K. G., Finley D. A., Lonnerdal B., 'Breast milk volume and composition during late lactation (7–20 months)'. *Journal of Pediatric Gastroenterology and Nutrition* 3(5) (Nov, 1984): 713–20.

Dewey K.G., Lonnerdal B., 'Milk and nutrient intake of breast-fed infants from 1 to 6 months: relation to growth and fatness'. *Journal of Pediatric Gastroenterology and Nutrition* 2(3) (1983): 497–506.

Dewey K. G., Heinig M. J., Nommsen L. A., Lonnerdal B., 'Maternal versus infant factors related to breast milk intake and residual milk volume: the DARLING study'. *Pediatrics* 87(6) (Jun, 1991): 829–37.

Bravi F, Wiens F, Decarli A, Dal Pont A, Agostoni C, Ferraroni M. Impact of maternal nutrition on breast-milk composition: a systematic review. *Am J Clin Nutr*. 2016;104(3):824–832. doi: 10.3945/ajcn.115.120881. PMID: 27534637.

Geddes D. T., Sakalidis V. S., 'The physiology of milk removal: Understanding the importance of frequent breast emptying for milk supply maintenance'. *Journal of Human Lactation*. 32(2) (2016): 280–290.

Kent J. C., Mitoulas L., Cox D. B., Owens R. A., Hartmann P. E., 'Breast volume and milk production during extended lactation in women'. *Experimental Physiology* 84(2) (Mar, 1999): 435–47.

Kim SY, Yi DY. Components of human breast milk: from macronutrient to microbiome and microRNA. *Clin Exp Pediatr*. 2020 Mar 23;63(8):301–309. doi: 10.3345/cep.2020.00059. PMCID: PMC7402982. PMID: 32252145.

La Leche League International. *The Womanly Art of Breastfeeding*. 8th ed. Schaumburg, IL: La Leche League International; 2010. Printed by Pinter & Martin Ltd.

McClellan H. L., Miller S. J., Hartmann P. E., 'Evolution of lactation: nutrition v. protection with special reference to five mammalian species'. *Nutrition Research Reviews*. 21(2) (Dec, 2008): 97–116.

EFSA Panel on Dietetic Products, Nutrition, and Allergies (NDA). Scientific Opinion on Dietary Reference Values for water. *EFSA J*. 2010 Mar 25;8(3):1459. doi: 10.2903/j.efsa.2010.1459.

Neville M. C., 'Studies in human lactation: Milk volumes in lactating women during the onset of lactation and full lactation'. *American Journal of Clinical Nutrition* 48(6) (Dec 1988): 1375–86.

Salazar G., Vio F., Garcia C., Aguirre E., Coward W. A. 'Energy requirements in Chilean infants'. *Archives of Disease in Childhood. Fetal Neonatal Ed* 83(2) (Sep, 2000): F120–3.

Chapter Five: Nurturing Yourself

Geddes L. Antibodies in breast milk remain for 10 months after Covid infection – study. *The Guardian*. 2021 Sep 27. Available from: https://www.theguardian.com/lifeandstyle/2021/sep/27/antibodies-in-breast-milk-remain-for-10-months-after-covid-infection-study

Collaborative Group on Hormonal Factors in Breast Cancer. Breast cancer and breastfeeding. *Lancet*. 2002;360(9328):187–195.

Deoni S.C., et al. Breastfeeding and early white matter development: A cross-sectional study. *NeuroImage*. 2013;82:77–86. DOI: 10.1016/j.neuroimage.2013.04.073.

Kendall-Tackett K.A. Depression in New Mothers: Causes, Consequences, and Treatment Alternatives. 3rd ed. New York: Routledge; 2016.

Moore E. R., Bergman N., Anderson G. C., Medley N., 'Early skin-to-skin contact for mothers and their healthy newborn infants'. *Cochrane Database of Systematic Reviews* 11(11) (2016): CD003519.

Chapter Six: Fuelling Your Breastfeeding

National Institutes of Health (NIH). When breastfeeding, how many calories should moms and babies consume? Available from: https://www.nichd.nih.gov/health/topics/breastfeeding/conditioninfo/calories.

Chapter Nine: Breastfeeding, Menstruation, Fertility and Pregnancy

Labbok M., 'Breastfeeding during pregnancy and risk of miscarriage: A systematic review'. *Perspectives on Sexual and Reproductive Health.* 51(3) (2019):143–150. https://www.guttmacher.org/journals/psrh/2019/09/breast-feeding-during-pregnancy-and-risk-miscarriage

Chapter Ten: How to Stop Breastfeeding

National Health Service (NHS). What to feed your baby: 10 to 12 months. https://www.nhs.uk/start-for-life/baby/weaning/what-to-feed-your-baby/10-to-12-months

National Health Service (NHS). What to feed your baby: Over 12 months. https://www.nhs.uk/start-for-life/baby/weaning/what-to-feed-your-baby/over-12-months

South West Yorkshire Partnership NHS Foundation Trust. Weaning and complementary feeding leaflet. https://www.southwestyorkshire.nhs.uk/wp-content/uploads/2020/09/Weaning-and-complementary-feeding-leaflet.pdf

Chapter Eleven: Celebrating Your Breastfeeding Journey

NHS Digital. Infant Feeding Survey – 2010, Early Results. https://digital.nhs.uk/data-and-information/publications/statistical/infant-feeding-survey/infant-feeding-survey-2010-early-results

Resources

Back to Work and Breastfeeding

- Acas – Acas provides guidance on breastfeeding rights at work, including workplace accommodations and legal protections.
  Website: www.acas.org.uk

Support for Postnatal Mental Health

- The Lullaby Trust – The most up-to-date research and guidelines on safe sleep and co-sleeping.
  Website: www.lullabytrust.org.uk

- Cry-sis – Support for parents dealing with excessive crying, colic and sleep issues in infants.
  Helpline: Helpline: 0800 448 0737
  Website: www.cry-sis.org.uk

- Mind – Postnatal Depression Support
  Information and support for postnatal depression, anxiety and perinatal mental health.
  Website: www.mind.org.uk

- PANDAS Foundation – Perinatal mental health support for parents struggling with anxiety or depression.
  Website: www.pandasfoundation.org.uk

Breastfeeding Support

- The Breastfeeding Network – Independent, evidence-based information and peer support for breastfeeding families.
  Website: www.breastfeedingnetwork.org.uk

- Association of Breastfeeding Mothers (ABM) – Practical breastfeeding support and helplines.
  Website: www.abm.me.uk
- La Leche League GB – Breastfeeding support groups and online help from trained breastfeeding counsellors.
  Website: www.laleche.org.uk
- *The Womanly Art of Breastfeeding* – A comprehensive book by La Leche League on breastfeeding and overcoming challenges. Available on Amazon or at local bookstores.

Infant Feeding and Health

- NHS – Tongue-tie information and support with NHS guide on identifying and treating tongue-ties in infants.
  Website: www.nhs.uk/conditions/tongue-tie
- NHS – Colic information and resources with NHS advice on symptoms, causes and managing colic in babies.
  Website: www.nhs.uk/conditions/colic
- NHS – Infant feeding guide with reliable information on breast-feeding, formula feeding and weaning.
  Website: www.nhs.uk/start-for-life

Scientific and Research-based Resources

Nguyen V. V. T., Zheng M. Y., Liu S. M., Kallen M. A., Kay K., Ivey S. L., 'Prevalence of traditional Asian postpartum practices at a federally qualified health center'. *Journal of Immigration and Minority Health*. 24(5) (Oct, 2022):1251–1260. doi: 10.1007/s10903-021-01299-0.

Segura-Bernal O., Muñoz-Lopez M., Ruiz-Aguilar F., Esparza-Reséndiz N., Arzate-Mejía R., Valverde-Estrella L., et al. Beyond nutrition: A review of the influence of early life breastfeeding on epigenetic programming of health and disease. *Front Nutr*. 2021;8:798974. DOI: 10.3389/fnut.2021.798974.

Glossary

A

Alzheimer's – A progressive disease that affects the brain, leading to memory loss, confusion and changes in behaviour. It is the most common cause of dementia.

B

Baby-wearing – The practice of carrying a baby in a sling or carrier, allowing for close contact between parent and child while keeping hands free.

Blocked Duct – A condition where a milk duct becomes clogged, causing discomfort and sometimes leading to mastitis if untreated.

Breastfeeding Aversion and Agitation (BAA) – A condition where a mother feels irritated, distressed or anxious while breastfeeding, even though she may normally enjoy it. This can sometimes be triggered by hormonal changes or stress.

C

Cardiac Vagal Tone – A measure of the activity of the vagus nerve that regulates heart rate and helps maintain a calm and relaxed state. It plays an important role in the body's stress response and emotional regulation.

Caesarean – A surgical procedure used to deliver a baby through incisions made in the mother's lower stomach and uterus, typically when a vaginal birth would pose a risk to the mother or baby.

Cessation – The process of stopping something; in this context, referring to the end of breastfeeding.

Chestfeeding – A term used to describe breastfeeding or human milk feeding by trans and non-binary parents who do not identify with the term 'breastfeeding'.

Choline – A vital nutrient important for brain development, particularly for infants and during pregnancy. Found in foods such as eggs, meat and fish.

Colic – A condition in which a baby experiences excessive, often unexplained crying, typically in the first few months of life.

Cortisol – A hormone released in response to stress, which can impact milk supply and infant sleep patterns.

D

Dysphoric Milk Ejection Reflex (D-MER) – A condition in which a mother experiences feelings of sadness, anxiety or irritability during milk let-down, even though she enjoys breastfeeding overall. These feelings are typically brief and go away as the milk flow starts.

E

Express Milk – The act of extracting milk from the breast using hand expression or a breast pump.

F

Freezer Stash – A supply of expressed breast milk stored in the freezer for future use.

Frenectomy/Frenotomy – Surgical procedures used to release or trim a tongue-tie or lip-tie, which are conditions where the frenulum (the piece of tissue that connects the tongue or lip to the mouth) is too tight, restricting movement. The tissue is cut using a surgical grade blade or a laser.

G

Ghrelin – A hormone that stimulates appetite and helps regulate hunger signals. It is sometimes referred to as the 'hunger hormone'.

H

Hypoplasia – A condition where there is an underdevelopment or incomplete development of a tissue or organ, such as in the case of insufficient glandular tissue in the breasts.

I

IBCLC (International Board Certified Lactation Consultant) – A healthcare professional who specialises in breastfeeding support and lactation care.

L

Lactation – The process of producing and secreting milk from the mammary glands.

Lactational Amenorrhoea – The absence of menstruation due to breastfeeding. This can occur as a natural contraceptive effect for some women in the early months of breastfeeding.

Lactocytes – The cells in the mammary glands that are responsible for producing milk.

Let-down – The reflex that causes breast milk to flow from the milk ducts to the nipple in response to a baby's suckling or other stimuli.

M

Macrophages – A type of white blood cell that helps fight infection by engulfing harmful bacteria, viruses and debris. They are present in breast milk and provide immune support to infants.

Mastitis – Inflammation of the breast, usually caused by a blocked duct or infection, often leading to pain, swelling and flu-like symptoms.

Matrescence – The transition to motherhood, encompassing the physical, emotional and psychological changes that occur.

Melatonin – A hormone that regulates sleep patterns, found in breast milk and contributing to infant circadian rhythm development.

Microchimerism – The presence of a small number of cells from another individual in the body, typically transferred during pregnancy. This can include cells from the mother in the child or vice versa.

Milk Shells – Devices worn inside a bra to collect leaking breast milk.

Milk Supply – The amount of breast milk a mother produces, influenced by factors such as demand, hydration and hormonal balance.

N

Nursing Strike – A sudden refusal by a baby to breastfeed, often temporary and caused by teething, illness or changes in routine.

O

Osteopathy – A form of complementary therapy that focuses on the structure and function of the body, sometimes used to help babies with feeding difficulties.

Osteoporosis – A condition where bones become weak and brittle, increasing the risk of fractures. It can be related to hormonal changes, such as those during menopause or breastfeeding.

Oxytocin – A hormone responsible for triggering the let-down reflex during breastfeeding and promoting bonding between mother and baby.

P

Paced Bottle Feeding – A feeding technique designed to mimic breastfeeding, allowing the baby to control the flow of milk and reducing the risk of overfeeding.

Parasympathetic – Part of the autonomic nervous system responsible for calming the body after stress. It promotes relaxation and recovery, often referred to as the 'rest and digest' system.

Parental Leave – A period of leave from work for parents following the birth or adoption of a child, allowing time to care for the child.

Postnatal Depression (PND) – A form of depression that affects parents after childbirth, often linked to hormonal changes, sleep deprivation and emotional adjustments.

Postpartum – The period following childbirth, often used interchangeably with 'postnatal' in British English.

Prolactin – A hormone responsible for milk production, stimulated by breastfeeding.

R

Rainbow Baby – A baby born after the loss of a previous pregnancy or infant, symbolising hope and healing.

Relaxin – A hormone produced during pregnancy and breastfeeding that increases joint flexibility, sometimes contributing to aches and pains.

Reverse Cycling – A pattern where a baby breastfeeds more frequently at night and less during the day, often occurring when a mother returns to work.

S

Silver Cups – Small silver nipple covers used to help heal sore or cracked nipples naturally.

Sleep Apnoea – A sleep disorder where breathing repeatedly stops and starts during sleep, leading to poor sleep quality and potential health issues.

Statutory Right – A legally protected right, such as the right to request flexible working arrangements or time to express milk in the workplace.

T

Teat – The rubber or silicone part of a bottle that a baby sucks on to drink milk or formula.

Teething – The process of a baby's teeth emerging through the gums, often causing discomfort and increased nursing for soothing.

Thrush – A fungal infection caused by candida yeast, which can develop in a baby's mouth or on a breastfeeding mother's nipples, leading to pain and discomfort.

V

Vagus Nerve – A long nerve that runs from the brainstem through the neck and chest to the abdomen. It plays a key role in regulating many bodily functions, including heart rate, digestion and respiratory rate.

Vestibular System – The sensory system responsible for balance and spatial awareness, which is developed through movement, baby-wearing and rocking.

Index

Note: Page numbers in italics refer to information contained in tables

adaptability 67–73
advice, unsolicited 200–4
affirmations 290, 296
alcohol consumption 187–90, 211
allergies 21, 61, 130, 136
alertness 44
Alzheimer's disease 19
amenorrhoea, lactational 250
antibiotics 151, 158, 159
antibodies 21, 201, 288
antifungal medications 153–4
anxiety 7–8, 61, 63–4, 80, 143, 147–8, 154, 175, 194
appetite 119–20
apps, baby-tracking 47–9
ARA (arachidonic acid) 20
attachment 21–2, 59, 176

baby loss 3–4, 8–9, 105
baby massage 131–2
baby-wearing 190–2
batch cooking 209
baths, Epsom salt 194
bedtimes 242–3, 276–7
beginning breastfeeding 17–40
   first six weeks 43–5
   benefits of breastfeeding 17–23

birth
   preparation for while breastfeeding 256–7
   traumatic 2–3, 8, 26, 105, 127
biting 139–40
blood sugar 121, 152, 213, 282
body, maternal 55, 65
bodywork
   for babies 127
   see also massage
bonding 21–2, 54, 59, 176, 258–9, 263, 288, 292–3
bone health 19
bottles
   delayed introduction 86
   introduction 278
   paced feeding 233–4, 237, 278
   refusal 237–40
boundaries
   breastfeeding 253–4, 256, 260, 267–8, 271, 277–9
   relationship 182, 196, 203, 223–6, 229–30
brain
   development 20, 201
   maternal 40, 56, 176
bras 101, 151, 198–9

breast cancer 18, 200
breast compression 85
'breast crawl' 25
'breast is best' 5
breast massage 99–100, 116, 144, 159, 166
breast milk
  analgesic content 138, 200
  benefits for baby 20–3
  freezer stashes 235, 237, 240–1, 245
  leakage 95, 101, 199, 241
  nutrients 20, 23, 200, 206–7, 258
  sensitivity to/intolerance of 130
  storage at work 232
  water content 117
  see also milk supply
breast refusal 140–4
breast surgery/trauma 89
Breastfeeding Aversion and Agitation (BAA) 167–70, 253, 259–61, 266
  see also Dysphoric Milk Ejection Reflex
breastfeeding journey, celebration 53, 55, 68, 106–8, 285–97
breastfeeding mechanisms 23–5
breastfeeding rates 12, 32, 216
breasts 76
  caring for 198–9
  engorgement 81, 95, 101, 245, 259, 263
  offering both 78–80, 85
  size 58
breathwork 37–8, 116, 177–80, 197
burping babies 100, 131, 136

Caesarean section 26, 27, 105
caffeine 211
calcium 207, 251, 255
calorie-requirements 119, 186, 206
cancer 18, 200
candida albicans 149
  see also nipple thrush
carbohydrates, complex 212
cardiac vagal tone 175
cardiovascular health 18–19
challenges, acknowledging 55–6
children's needs 68, 177–81, 184
cholecystokinin (CCK) 110
choline 162, 166–7, 211
circadian rhythms 65–6, 110
clothing 136, 155, 166
cluster feeds 44, 62, 103–4, 216
co-sleeping 50
colic 126, 128–33
colostrum 3, 27, 254–5
combination feeding 5–6, 84, 235–6, 286
comfort associations, layering 275–7
communication skills 221, 229–30, 275
community support 87
compassion 204
  see also self-compassion
compresses
  cold 101, 161
  warm 161, 166
concentration 197–8
confinement periods 54
contraception 251
cortisol 66, 110, 118, 145, 175

cranial osteopathy 79, 127
Cry-sis 133
crying babies 44, 128–9, 132

dancing 185
day and night, establishing patterns of 65–6
dehydration 118, 212
depression 147–8
  postnatal 12, 80, 176–7, 195, 269–70
development 20, 201, 242
DHA (docosahexaenoic acid) 20, 207
diet 93, 119–22, 191, 206–14
  and breastfeeding when pregnant 251, 255–6
  elimination 131–2, 136
  foods to prioritise/avoid 211
  sugary foods 152–3
  and weaning 282–3
distraction techniques 272–3
domperidone 84
donor milk 5, 84, 227, 235–6, 286
ducts, clogged 80, 95, 101, 105–6, 126, 143–4, 156–60
dummies 86
Dysphoric Milk Ejection Reflex (D-MER) 24, 118, 169, 170

elimination diets 131–2, 136
emotions 221, 227–8, 253
  and breastfeeding 174–5, 177
  and clogged ducts/mastitis 159–60
  and nursing aversion 168, 169–70
  and weaning 261, 269–70, 272, 279–80, 280–4
endorphins 200
energy levels 65, 121, 212
engorgement 81, 95, 101, 245, 259, 263
enlightenment 198
Epsom salt baths 194
exhaustion 7, 33, 36, 38–9, 41, 47–8, 52, 56, 60–1, 103–4, 108, 137, 148, 173, 194, 197, 213, 216, 242, 253, 261, 266–7, 293
expectations 1–2, 221
expressing
  and breast refusal 142
  and establishing a milk supply 28
  and labelling milk 110
  and returning to work 230, 234–7, 245
extended breastfeeding 288–9
eye movements, rapid 45

failure, feelings of 2, 4, 11–12, 60–1, 87
family relationships 223, 224–5
'fed is best' 5
feeding
  amounts 63–4
  baby-led 58–9
  block 96
  combination 5–6, 84, 235–6, 286
  on demand 1–3, 36, 45–6, 52, 59–61, 83, 85, 92, 168, 189, 203, 223, 250, 266, 272
  frequency 45–7, 46, 58–9, 81, 85, 91, 126, 136

Index • 315

feeding – *cont.*
  gaps between 85
  logs/diaries 62–5, 77
  long feeds 43, 126
  and managing milk supply 74–122
  night-time 49–50, 59–62, 85, 243, 265–6
  normal 45–7, *46*
  one-sided 78–9, 96
  pacing 101
  patterns of 45–7, *46*, 62
  routines 62–5
  triple 83–4
  turn-taking with 50–1
  unsatisfying 76, 78, 80
  see also cluster feeds; night-feeding; stopping breastfeeding
feeding apps 47–9
fertility 90, 105, 249, 251
flexibility 41–3, 62–5, 72, 180–4
food allergies/sensitivities 136
food cravings 212–13
formula milk 5–6, 84, 278, 286
  the 'formula trap' 28
  how to introduce 236
fourth trimester *see* post-partum period
frenectomy/frenotomy 29, 127
friendships 223–5, 230
fussiness 44, 91, 92, 129, 150

gas 126, 129, 130, 131
ghrelin 119
'Golden Hour' 25–6
grace, giving yourself 52–3
gratitude practice 56
grounding 178–9

growth spurts 81, 90–4, 242
gut health 21, 22, 153

help, asking for 35, 64–5, 86–7, 102, 128, 132–3, 137, 155–6, 159, 162–3, 167, 170–1, 193, 208, 256–7, 296–7
hormonal changes 119–20, 124, 152, 169, 219–20, 253, 269–70, 280–2
hormonal feedback loops 27, 124
hormonal imbalance 88–90
household chores 51, 147, 192
hunger cues 43–5
hydration 93, 101, 116, 117–19, 121, 147, 159, 186–7, 212, 251, 282
  see also water intake
hygiene practice 153, 154–5

illness 90, 141
immune system 20–2, 120–1, 151–2, 200–1, 288
infertility 90, 105
instinct, trusting your 81–2
insufficient glandular tissue (IGT) 89–90
internal working model 181–2
International Board Certified Lactation Consultant (IBCLC) 10–11, 25, 32, 75, 77, 82, 86, 89, 96, 102, 126–7, 131
intimacy 215, 217–22
iron, dietary 255

jewellery, breast milk 286
journalling 38–40, 55–8, 106–8, 182–4, 228–30, 262, 283, 294–6

keeping up appearances 42–3
kefir-based products 283

lactocytes 23, 58
latches
 and biting 139
 checking 28, 31–2, 77
 and colic 130–1
 deep 139
 good 29–32
 and low milk supply 82
 and nipple shields 140
 optimisation 82
 and oral ties 125–7
 poor 130–1, 136, 150, 153–4
 and Raynaud's syndrome 166
 and reflux 136
 shallow 125–6
 and thrush 150, 153–4
lecithin 162, 166–7
let-down reflex 124
 and alcohol consumption 189
 forceful 81, 94, 95, 101, 130, 131, 133–5
 management 98–9
letter-writing 291–4
libido 219–20
lip smacking 44
lip-ties 124–8
Lullaby Trust 50

magnesium 194, 251, 255
massage 99–100, 116, 131–2, 144, 159, 166
mastitis 80, 95, 101, 124, 126, 156–61
matrescence 7, 193
'me-time' 180–1, 183, 193
meal planning 208–10

meditation 147–8, 198, 294–6
melatonin 66, 110
menstrual cycle 249–51
mental health 4, 12, 33, 35, 48–9, 80, 86–7, 176–7, 182, 189–90, 195, 269–70
microchimerism 9
milk blebs 160–3
milk catchers 111
milk flow 100–1, 124
milk shells 241
milk supply
 and breast care 198–9
 and breast refusal 141–2
 changes over time 74–5, 141–2
 and diet 206–14
 during pregnancy 254–6
 establishing 42, 43–4, 54, 58
 and growth spurts 90–4
 low supply 12, 28, 75–90, 106
  causes 88–90
  identification 76
  management 82–6
  and mental health 86–7
  perceived low 74, 77–82
  steps to take 77
  true low 74, 77–90
 management 74–122
 and the menstrual cycle 250–1
 and night feeding 59
 oversupply 75–6, 81, 94–102
  and colic 130, 131
  gidentification 95
  management 96–102
  and pumping 111
  and reflux 133–5
  signs of 95, 101

milk supply – *cont.*
  and pumping 83–4, 85–6, 90, 94, 98–102
  and sleep 32–3, 36
  supporting 26–32, 59, 62, 121
  and tandem feeding 258–9, 261, 263
  and work trips 245
  mindfulness 69–73, 177–80, 198
miscarriage 3–4, 8–9, 105
motherhood 294–7
  journey of 292
  reflection on the meaning of 57
  transition to 6–7, 193
  undervaluing of 53–5
  see also newborns, adjusting to life with
mothers, caring for new 54–5
multiples 258
music 116–17, 184–5

nappies 51, 76
nappy rash 150, 156
naps 65
nature, spending time in 34, 185–6, 282
neural pruning 40
newborns 21, 25–6, 27–8
  adjusting to life with 41–73
  needs 68
  stomach size 27, 41–2
  and tandem feeding 249, 256, 257–64
night-feeding 49–50, 59–62, 85, 243, 265–6
night-waking 60–2, 69
nipple shields 140
nipple thrush 31, 149–56

nipples
  and biting 140
  blanching 163–7
  and breast pumps 116
  cracked 124–5, 151, 155
  and latches 30
  and oral ties 124–5
  painful 12, 31, 124–5, 140, 149–50, 154–6, 258
  shape after feeding 31
  soaking in warm water 161
  and tandem feeding 258
niyama 196–7
noise sensitivity 185
nursing strikes 140–4
nurture 21–2, 292

oestrogen 88, 119–20, 253, 281
open cups 239
oral exams, manual 127
oral thrush 22, 150–1, 153–4
oral ties 29, 124–8, 135
osteoporosis 19
ovarian cancer 18
overstimulation
  and babies 131, 141–2
  and milk supply 99, 100
overwhelm 8, 11, 14, 33, 38, 41, 43, 45–6, 48, 63–4, 68, 81, 86, 103–4, 123, 133, 169, 177, 183, 253, 258, 263
ovulation 250, 251
oxytocin 19, 21, 23–5, 34, 65, 83, 116, 124, 175–7, 219, 244, 269–70, 280–1

pain relief 159, 162
pain when breastfeeding 25, 31–2, 169

and clogged ducts and mastitis 156–9, 161
and milk blebs 160–3
and oral ties 29, 124, 125
and Raynaud's syndrome 163–6
see also nipples, painful
patience 163
perfectionism 3, 210–11, 273
physical strain 69
placenta, delivery 26
polycystic ovary syndrome (PCOS) 8, 88–9
positioning baby 29–30, 77, 82, 97
    laid-back position 97
    and nipple thrush 155
    and oral ties 126–7
    and Raynaud's syndrome 166
    and reflux 136
    side-lying position 97, 98
postnatal depression 12, 80, 176–7, 195, 269–70
postpartum period 41–73, 138, 184, 194–7, 291
postpartum psychosis 48–9
pregnancy
    breastfeeding during 249, 251–7, 260–2, 264
    reflection on 56
probiotics 153
progesterone 26, 88, 119–20, 253
prolactin 19, 23–4, 26–7, 33, 84, 88, 118, 124, 219, 250, 269–70, 280–1
protein 120–1, 207, 212–13
psychosis, postpartum 48–9
public breastfeeding 200
pumping 1, 2, 5–6, 74–5, 79, 98–122, 286, 291–2

and cluster feeds 103–4
and combination feeding 84
and diet 119–22
emotional demands of 103, 104–6
and journalling 106–8
managing 109–19, 121–2
and milk supply 83–4, 85–6, 90, 94, 98–102
parallel 241
physical demands of 103, 104–6
and rest 103–4
and returning to work 227, 230–3, 235, 237, 240–1, 245
rewards of 109
rhythm of 103–4
time requirements 106
tips 116–17
and triple feeding 83–4
and turn-taking 50–1
pumps 83, 110–17

Raynaud's syndrome 163–7
reflux 126, 133–8
relationships 214, 215–26
relaxin 195–6
rest 32–5, 39, 51–2, 93, 183
    at the same time as baby 147
    and clogged ducts/mastitis 159
    and milk blebs 163
    and pumping 103–4
retained products of conception (RPOC) 88
reverse cycling 241–3
rhythm, finding a 41–73, 103–4
romantic relationships 215–22
rooting reflex 44

self-care 34, 35, 54–5, 57, 61, 143, 155, 163, 171, 172–205
  modelling for the next generation 181–2, 184
self-compassion 53, 72, 87, 128, 204–5, 252, 257, 295
self-kindness 148, 196, 280
self-love 110, 295
separation anxiety 7–8, 143
serotonin 194
settling babies 51
shared parenting 192–3, 243
sibling rivalry 257–8, 259
silicone suction breast pumps 112
silver cups 140
sippy cups 239
skin-to-skin contact 21, 25–6, 83, 142, 176, 192, 275
sleep
  baby's 91–2, 144–9, 245–6
  and growth spurts 91, 92
  maternal naps 65
  prioritising your 32–3
  shift-pattern schedules 50
  sleep deprivation 3, 6, 11, 36–8, 42, 47–8, 60–2, 134, 148
sleep disruption
  in babies 144–9
  and stopping breastfeeding 269, 281–2
sleep hormones 110
sleep stories 276–7
sleep-training 8, 144–6
'slowing down' 33
snacks 116, 120–2, 208, 210, 212, 282
soothing/calming techniques 131–2, 142–3

sphincter muscles, immature 135
spitting up 134–5
stopping breastfeeding
  see weaning
stress 36, 61, 81, 118, 166, 175
stretching 194–6
sucking 30, 44
  suck-training exercises 127
Sudden Infant Death Syndrome (SIDS) 60
sugar intake 152–3
supplemental nursing system (SNS) 84
swallowing 30
  air 126, 130–1, 135
  sounds 76
switch nursing 85

tandem breastfeeding 249, 256, 257–64
teething 138–40, 141
tension, relief 38, 69–72, 93–4, 127, 194
thoughts, intrusive 48–9
thyroid hormones 88–9
time with your child 242, 244
tongue-ties 29, 124–8
'touched out', feeling 169, 183, 219–20, 266
troubleshooting 123–71
tummy massage 131, 132

visualisation 35
vitamins 207, 255, 255–6
vomiting 134, 137

walking 34–5
water intake 279
  see also hydration

weaning 12, 124, 246, 253–4, 261, 264, 265–84, 289–90
  abrupt 246, 269–70, 272
  ceremonies/traditions 286–8
  child-led 261, 270–1, 273
  gentle 274–80
  giving yourself permission 274
  and the last feed 268, 280
  parent-led 261, 265–8, 271–4
  premature 17, 227, 246, 249
  as process 273–4
'weaning blues' 269, 281–4
weight gain 63, 76–7, 91, 96
work trips 244–7
work-life balance 229
working mothers 7, 34, 124, 227–48
  babies over six months 236–8
  babies under six months 234–6
  preparing babies 233–4, 247
  workplace policies and rights 230–1
World Health Organization (WHO) 3

yama 4, 69, 196
yoga 4, 69–73, 194–8
  asanas 70–2, 196
  Cat-Cow Stretch 70
  dharana 197–8
  Eight Limbs of 196–8
  pranayama 37–8, 197
  pratyahara 197
  Reclining Bound Angle Pose 71, 72
  Seated Forward Bend 70–1
  Sphinx Pose 71–2

zinc 207

About the Author

Danielle Facey, also known as 'The Breastfeeding Mentor', is a dedicated advocate for breastfeeding, maternal wellness and mental health. A trained Breastfeeding Counsellor with a Master's degree in Psychology, Danielle brings both professional expertise and lived experience to her work. Her passion for supporting nursing mothers began with her own journey – navigating the joys and challenges of breastfeeding through infancy, returning to work and extended nursing in a society that often lacks understanding and support.

A former English teacher, Danielle's love of language and storytelling shines through in her work, making her guidance both accessible and empowering. She believes deeply that maternal mental health and a child's well-being are not opposing forces but rather elements of a beautiful, symbiotic relationship – one that deserves to be nurtured and celebrated.

Through her social media channels, Danielle has built a thriving global community of over 275,000 mothers, offering encouragement, evidence-based advice and a much-needed voice of solidarity. When she isn't mentoring and supporting parents, she enjoys practising yoga and meditation – both of which inform her holistic approach to maternal well-being. She's also a keen walker, reader and baker. She lives in Birmingham with the love of her life and their son, both of whom inspire her daily.